## PRAISE FOR BETTER BODY BOOTCAMP

Three hours a week at BBB will melt the fat ri‌ ‍
body. It did for me, and faster than you ‍
Within my first three months, I was ‍
jeans, lost significant body fat, and no‍ ‍ ‍ng
and reshaping in a way that has never be‍ ‍ possible.
RESULTS! And that was only coming three times a week. Now
I come four or five times a week because I love the way it
makes me feel. I get to work out with the greatest group of
people and get skinny all at once.

**—Jamie Jensen**

Going in, I was already a bit pessimistic because of my
previous unsuccessful attempts to lose weight. I had been
to several gyms and had gone on many diets, but something
about BBB made me feel strong and determined from the
minute I walked in. The truth is that no matter where you go,
you have to work hard and give it all you've got. But the difference between BBB and other gyms is that BBB makes it fun
to work out. Thank you, BBB, for believing in me and making
me believe in myself! I'm more confident than ever before.
You have changed my whole life!

**—Anna Konstandinidis**

This is the best gym ever! Excellent instructors. No two workout classes are ever the same. You are always pushed to your max and then some. The social climate is friendly and supportive. If you want to break through plateaus and reach high toward your full athletic potential, this is the place to go!

**—Neesa Suncheuri**

Love, love, love it! After all these years and lots of money down the drain, I found a gym I love and am sticking to. Thanks for helping this old Stella get her groove back!

**—Stella Vlamis Pappas**

Joining BBB almost two years ago was the best decision I have ever made regarding my fitness! The classes are always changing and always challenging. The trainers are amazing, and the place is like a family. I am addicted and cannot imagine working out anywhere else ever again! I wake up every day thinking about the next workout!

**—Helen Jones**

I instantly connected with the family atmosphere that BBB produces and the passion and drive that the trainers have. I can't help but smile when I walk into BBB knowing how much it has impacted my life already. I am looking forward to continuing my classes and seeing where it takes me.

**—Elliot Kleinburd**

CHANGE YOUR BODY AND LIFE IN **30 DAYS**

# BETTER BODY BOOT CAMP

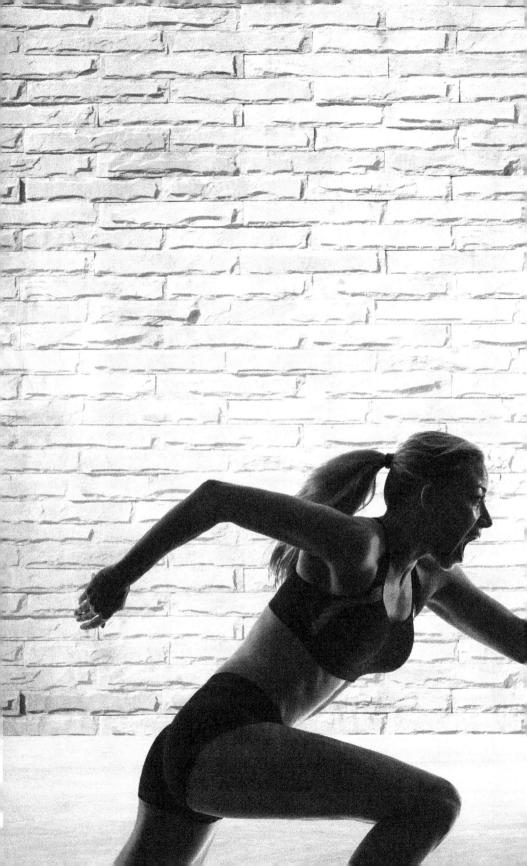

CHANGE YOUR BODY AND LIFE IN **30 DAYS**

# BETTER BODY BOOT CAMP

THE REVOLUTIONARY APPROACH FOR
**THE BODY AND LIFE YOU DESERVE**

★★★★★★★★★★★★★★★★★★★★★★★★★★★★★★★★★★

# KAISER SERAJUDDIN

*Advantage*®

Published by Advantage, Charleston, South Carolina.
Member of Advantage Media Group.

ADVANTAGE is a registered trademark, and the Advantage colophon is a trademark of Advantage Media Group, Inc.

Printed in the United States of America.

10  9  8  7  6  5  4  3  2  1

ISBN: 978-1-59932-833-1
LCCN: 2017956053

Cover and layout design by George Stevens.

This publication is designed to provide accurate and authoritative information in regard to the subject matter covered. It is sold with the understanding that the publisher is not engaged in rendering legal, accounting, or other professional services. If legal advice or other expert assistance is required, the services of a competent professional person should be sought.

Advantage Media Group is proud to be a part of the Tree Neutral® program. Tree Neutral offsets the number of trees consumed in the production and printing of this book by taking proactive steps such as planting trees in direct proportion to the number of trees used to print books. To learn more about Tree Neutral, please visit **www.treeneutral.com.**

Advantage Media Group is a publisher of business, self-improvement, and professional development books. We help entrepreneurs, business leaders, and professionals share their Stories, Passion, and Knowledge to help others Learn & Grow. Do you have a manuscript or book idea that you would like us to consider for publishing? Please visit advantagefamily.com or call **1.866.775.1696.**

*Dedicated to all of my clients, past and present.*

*It has been your belief in me that made me believe in myself, and it was your support that helped me achieve my dreams. I hope I was able to bring as much value to your lives as you have to mine.*

# FOREWORD

As a promoter of the numerous products that bear my name, I have the tremendous opportunity to talk with thousands of trainers and fitness business owners from around the world every year, from the trainers of the stars you see on TV and know by name, to the part-timers that are using Lebert EQualizer® and training a few clients in their driveway. But above the pack, there's one person that when he speaks, I listen, and that's Kaiser.

He's one of those guys that is not only involved in theory of how to motivate, achieve results, and create a revolution. He also puts his words into action. Through Better Body Bootcamp, I've observed firsthand the thousands of people he's helped, the amazing culture he's created, the lives he's transformed, and his tremendous business success. In the world of fitness, there's a lot of talk and a lot of pretenders. Anyone can write a book about getting in shape, and these days, just about everyone has. But it's unique when you've actually met someone that's molded as many people as Kaiser has through a completely new approach to fitness. An approach is only revolutionary if it achieves phenomenal real-world success. That's what I've seen Kaiser's program do firsthand.

My relationship with fitness is very similar to Kaiser's, and I see its power every day. Technology is killing us, and we are bombarded with so many crazy body-image and fast-food messages. It's no wonder we are where we are. Some of the things you hear in this book may not be the easiest pills to swallow. It's easier to listen to those who simply feed you what you want to hear: buy a fitness gadget to collect dust, continue with a yo-yo approach that doesn't work, or admit defeat and sit on the couch. While you're reading this book, you may feel uncomfortable with certain truths and automatically want to fight hard for your excuses. Don't. Allow yourself to hear the words and take them in with understanding and compassion for where you are at. As a trainer, I have seen many clients succeed because they were willing to accept new ideas and the feelings that come with them. Discomfort is there to let us know we may need to look at another path. Don't ignore it, but take that chance to see what new potential may exist for you.

Think about this for a moment: Movement is a very big part of the human condition. It's how we express our thoughts and feelings. Without it, we cannot realize much of what we think about. We build cities, dance with our partners, and break world records. This is because of movement. Studies have shown that getting out for a walk every day can be as powerful as any antidepressant, and as little as thirty minutes of physical activity can prevent adult onset diabetes. I have seen first-hand many cultures that bike to work and buy fresh food daily, and their incidence of heart disease and cancer is far less than ours. Something that we used to take so much joy in as children has become foreign to us, our culture, and the way we think. And the crazy thing is that it's not until you start to move again, to revel in its beauty, that you start to feel amazing once again.

I think that's what you'll find with this book. It will give you the motivation to move. After that, it will teach you how to harness this movement. Because these are real-world, tried-and-tested workout truths and not theory, you'll see the results for your efforts. Because of these immediate results, you'll hunger for more, and a feedback loop will be created and your life will be transformed.

You're in for an enjoyable read. Open your mind, and the rest will take care of itself.

**MARC LEBERT**

*Lebert International*
*Creator of the Lebert EQualizer®, used by trainers worldwide*

# ACKNOWLEDGMENTS

The book has been a project three years in the making, but it couldn't have come together at a better time. What finally pushed it over the edge to getting done? It's the unique and amazing mix of people that make up the fitness movement we call Better Body Bootcamp: the network of members, the BBB team, and an entire ecosystem of associates and influences that make Better Body possible.

Thanks to all those I just mentioned for your positive energy. It's my belief that what we're all pursuing in life, both inside of us and in our environment, is more positive energy. By creating strength, endurance, and improving your outward persona, you are nurturing the ability to produce even more positive energy. The effect this can have on the community and people is astounding. Better Body is proof of that, and this book is an extension of that.

First of all, credit goes to our incredible members. This wouldn't be possible without you, because you have been the case study for everything that this book is about. There isn't a warmer, more energetic, more generous, and more beautiful group of people that's ever come together.

Next is the Better Body Bootcamp team. I'm looking forward to many more years of growth with you as we get closer to achieving our goals and making a lasting difference. There's an invisible hand that has brought us all together, because a group like us could not have come together by accident.

Foremost credit goes to my mother, who gave me the space to find my interests and talents, and who has always believed in me to pursue them. You have never given me a wrong piece of advice in my life; it just took me time to understand all of it. And to my father, who showed me the value of hard work and discipline. Your passion and energy for work and achievement inspires me every day.

To my many mentors through the years: There's no Harvard for being a trainer, meaning there's no real guidance in this profession. For someone who wants to get to the top, there's only the mentorship of others. To my dozens of friends in the training industry, you have helped me shave years off of the learning curve and helped make BBB an overnight success.

In the worlds of fitness and business, and where they intersect to create a training business, there are giants both living and dead who provide daily inspiration. Thanks goes to you for showing us all what's possible. You are the true inspiration behind the Better Body mission: the realization of each of our own unlimited potential.

# TABLE OF CONTENTS

# A WORD FROM THE AUTHOR

When I first began my life as a fitness trainer, most everyone I knew thought I was nuts. To my family and classmates, switching my focus from working towards a medical degree to instead pursue a career as a personal trainer made about as much sense as diving off a cliff. Let's be honest: few parents run to call their friends and extended family to tell them their kid abandoned a doctorate degree to get a trainer's certificate. But I knew something big they didn't know at the time.

I understood very clearly that personal fitness was about much more than big muscles and skinny waists. More importantly, I knew that if I could just show others the impact fitness can have on people's physical and mental health and on their lives in general, then I could change the perception of not only personal trainers, but also of the fitness world as a whole. It was a lofty goal to be sure, but it gave me a profound sense of purpose when developing my own gym and fitness program, Better Body Bootcamp (BBB).

That sense of purpose, I reasoned, would be as vital to my business success as it would be to convincing my stunned parents that I hadn't lost my mind. To help put their concerns into perspective, you should know that my father worked for many years as a very high-level scientist in the pharmaceutical industry. He is now a tenured professor at a major university. My mom was also a professional in the same industry. What even they realized after learning more about the field I ultimately chose, however, was that if you approach training the right way, it too can save lives.

**If I could just show others the impact fitness can have on people's physical and mental health and on their lives in general, then I could change the perception of not only personal trainers but also of the fitness world as a whole.**

Today, BBB has three locations and counting across New York State and has served over ten thousand clients of every ability and experience level. For more than a decade, my trainers and I have watched thousands of lives change for the better by using the all-encompassing approach to fitness that our program employs. By motivating members to challenge what they have settled for, we have proven repeatedly that unlocking maximum physical potential offers more than just a great body. It restores, in the process, control over lifestyle, affording our members the confidence to reach for the kind of life they have always wanted: one of courage, vitality, happiness, and longevity.

This book serves as a summary of the knowledge I've gained along this journey. It's been nearly two decades in the making, inspired by a dedication to personal fitness and a seemingly insatiable appetite to learn more and push further than anyone in my industry ever has before. During that time, I've traveled the country, consulting with world-renowned trainers such as Gunnar Peterson, Tony Horton, Jake "Body by Jake" Steinfeld, and Todd Durkin. I've spent countless hours talking fitness and health with physicians, pharmacists, scientists, nutritionists, athletes, and everyday people from all walks of life in order to gain a deeper understanding of how fitness plays a role in our individual lives and the society around us.

**During that time, I've traveled the country, consulting with world-renowned trainers such as Gunnar Peterson, Tony Horton, Jake "Body by Jake" Steinfeld, and Todd Durkin.**

I included what I've learned in three sections within this book, each one representing a different stage in the fitness cycle. We begin with "Purpose," a collection of the various motives and environmental factors related to personal fitness. From the many ways your physical health affects your life to the societal pressures and common lifestyle hurdles you face, you will learn how a system that supports unhealthy living came into existence and what you can do to break out of it.

**I included what I've learned in three sections within this book, each one representing a different stage in the fitness cycle.**

By understanding the purposes and benefits of a fitter self, the motivation needed for creating real, long-lasting change will be all the easier to find if and when you lose your way. With a sense of purpose in hand, we will move on to "Sweat." As the name suggests, "Sweat" is dedicated to the hardest but most rewarding portion of personal fitness: the workout. In this section, you will find some of my favorite exercises, habits, and tools you can use to build a better body, as well as tips and advice on fostering an environment that supports a fitness lifestyle.

Lastly, we will explore topics on nutrition in the section, "Replenish." All the sweat, tears, blisters, and panting in the gym is minimized greatly if you aren't eating right. "Replenish" delves into the nutrients your body needs and how they're used, the foods you need to avoid, and the concept of nutrient timing, and provides an overview of the science behind your body's relationship with food.

These sections form a book that's structured in the same way your fitness routine should be: you begin each workout with a purpose or goal in mind for that day, execute it, restore your body with the proper nutrients, and then do it again. Perhaps a motto is in order. As we like to say here at BBB: "Eat, sleep, BBB, repeat!" Now, let's get to it!

# 1

# PURPOSE

# CHAPTER 1

# MORE THAN JUST LOOKS

**F**itness is the most important part of your life. That's not hype. I don't say that as hyperbole to sell you a treadmill or diet supplements. Fitness should be your top priority every single day. I know what you may be thinking, and honestly, I don't blame you. On the surface, fitness sounds more like vanity than it does an all-important feature of your life. But fitness is much more than the way you look; it will affect every area of your life, from your career, to your relationships, to your health. That means your fitness level will actually determine the very way you live your life. Look at it this way: The *purpose* of fitness is to improve your quality of life; looking good is simply a bonus. Don't believe me? Let's take a step back, and I'll prove it to you.

For as long as most of us can remember, fitness has been presented to the public all wrong. It was either about slimming down or bulking up, and it's mostly been sold to us through equipment and exercise programs that target only a few key glamour muscles and use a revolving door of well-marketed gimmicks. So, it's not your fault if you don't believe me when I say that fitness has an effect on every part of your life. In fact, many people ignore fitness altogether because they think its scope is actually quite limited. According to the Centers for Disease Control and Prevention (CDC), 78.3 percent of adults over the age of eighteen do not meet the CDC's physical activity guidelines for strength and aerobic activity. Those who do join a gym, buy a piece of equipment, or decide to start exercising usually do so with this mind-set: "Hey, maybe I'll wear a size smaller. Maybe the notch on my belt is going to be a little lower. Maybe when I take my clothes off, I'll feel a little more confident. Maybe I'll have a little more energy in a day." I probably don't need to tell you how far that mind-set will take you.

Fitness takes on a new level of importance when you learn, through the lens of science, about the effects of neglecting it. For years, scientific studies on sedentary lives have pointed to alarming findings. Unfortunately, they have gone largely unheard or ignored among a public that's increasingly unfazed by a daily deluge of bad news. It's one thing to hear that when you abandon, neglect, or never start a fitness regimen, you are not enjoying the benefits of having a better body. It's another thing altogether, however, when you hear from researchers that our physical and mental health suffers drastically from our lack of exercise and poor diet. No one enjoys hearing the news that our sex drive goes down as our anxiety levels go up, or that our ability to handle stress and resist bad foods and risky lifestyle choices is weakened by not working out. And we really don't want to hear that our risk of serious physical and psychological disease can increase from a minimum of 21 percent for some, all the way to 90 percent for others, just because of a lack of activity.[1]

We don't usually associate our fitness level with our sleep, social activities, relationships, hobbies, careers, mental fortitude, or our finances. That's not your fault, either. Fitness has typically been portrayed as either a new hobby to casually pick up or a vanity sport you have no time for, instead of the lifestyle overhaul that it is. Some of you may even be thinking along the same lines we trainers hear all the time: "It's mostly just genetics, right? I don't think I can get in shape, no matter how hard I work," or, "My doctor will probably have better news for me when I go see him. If not, then I'll just take a statin or whatever he'll prescribe for me and I'll be fine," or, "Sure, I'm depressed every now and then, but my mood probably doesn't have much to do with fitness. I'm just worried about other stuff. It will pass."

These are just excuses, and none of them are true. The idea that fitness is something only for jocks, models, and people with good genes and too much time on their hands is wrong. The rationale that it doesn't impact every other area of life outside personal appearance couldn't be further from the truth, either. It touches every aspect of your life in some major way, and in some ways, it's the defining factor in how you experience life.

Don't feel bad, though. I'm not judging or scolding you if you haven't gotten into fitness yet. I really can't say that I blame you.

---

1   Alisa Hrustic, "7 Surprising Ways You Wreck Your Body When You Don't Get Off Your Butt," *Men's Health*, March 1, 2017, accessed September 3, 2017, http://www.menshealth.com/health/effects-of-sedentary-lifestyle/slide/6

There aren't many legitimate solutions out there, and you may be just one of the hundreds of millions of people who haven't been fully motivated to get fit. Something you'll come to learn about me, though, is that while I will never blame you for ignorance or for the options you don't have, I won't let you off the hook for the knowledge and options you do have but ignore or reject. I hold all my clients just as responsible for the choices they make as I do the choices they don't make. And as I tell them, if you want in, you're responsible; if you want out, you're responsible.

> **That's what having a better body is all about. We're not just talking about looks here; we're talking about building a better, stronger, healthier life by first building a better, stronger, healthier body.**

My purpose as your "trainer-in-print" is to energize your drive to learn, grow, and transform your life by improving your body. As I tell everyone I meet, "As your body goes, so does your life." That's what having a better body is all about. We're not just talking about looks here; we're talking about building a better, stronger, healthier life by first building a better, stronger, healthier body.

So, with that spirit in mind, let me issue my first piece of tough love: It *is* your fault if you don't want to change. If you don't think you can treat your fitness with the seriousness it deserves, then this isn't the right book for you. To us at BBB, fitness is the connection between your time here on earth and the quality of that time. How much of your life that will be lived disease-free and able-bodied is directly related to how seriously you take your fitness. How you experience your life, the "happiness" you feel during that time in particular, has a great deal to do with your fitness level and the impact it has on your mind and body. To put it bluntly, without committing yourself to the seriousness of what you're about to pursue, you won't just fail at the BBB approach; you will fall well short of your best no matter which fitness approach you try.

Chances are you're reading this book after trying to get fit. Perhaps you've tried other programs already, listened to other trainers, or even read other books. Maybe you played sports in the past, or you've worked out on your own before, but you're new to training, or you've never done a single push-up or run a single lap around the track in your entire life—a true clean slate. Wherever you're starting from, let's try something new. Let's forget everything you may have heard, read, or seen about fitness and start afresh. Deal? Great, let's get started building your own better body then.

In the pages ahead, I'll show you the ideas behind building a Better Body by discussing:

★ **The Fitness Instinct**
★ **The Attraction Effect**
★ **Healthy Parenting**
★ **Financial Fitness**
★ **Body Over Mind**

## THE FITNESS INSTINCT

When we're talking about fitness, one thing you need to understand is that there is no activity more ingrained in our basic human instincts than fitness, especially the way we do it at BBB. Fitness is about sweating. It's about moving. It's about lifting. It's about strength. It's about survival. There is nothing more primal than that. These days, most of us sit in cars and on trains, at desks and tables, or on the couch for more hours than we do anything else. Most jobs don't involve physical labor at all, so there's nothing like physical fitness that hearkens back to our early days as roaming hunter-gatherer tribes.

Whatever our religious beliefs are, whether we think we were once all naked in a garden, evolved from fish, or fell out of a spaceship, we can all agree that life was once very different for our earliest ancestors. But even though the average life for us back then would have been a lot more primal than our lives today, many of our instincts and needs remain. We like to eat. We love sex. We love our friends and family, our tribe of sorts. We like to watch people punch each other's lights out, or crash into each other on the football field, or dominate each other on the basketball court, or do something else incredibly daring and difficult. Food, water, and shelter comprise our number-one priorities, but competition, the physical challenging of both ourselves and one another, is still a favorite of ours as well.

## THE ATTRACTION EFFECT

Fitness is going to have an almost animalistic impact on your life, igniting an invigorating, fundamental response that may surprise you. Take attraction, for instance. Not only is attraction the most common reason people want to get in shape; it's also fitness's strongest tie to our primal side. Whether we're actively single or we just want to impress our partner, physical attractiveness matters. That might not be the case in a perfect world, but in this world, we all judge people's overall attractiveness, to some degree, by their body and how it's functioning. In other words, the person you most want to sleep with is most likely a healthy person.

Attractiveness indicators are also indicators of fitness, all of which tell us something about our offspring's chances of survival. Waist-to-hip ratio in women, for example, is relative to the hips being important in childbearing. Today the waist-to-hip ratio is almost entirely influenced by your diet and fitness level. In men, the v-taper—meaning a man's shoulder-to-waist ratio—is considered desirable. Men and women with a poor shoulder-to-waist ratio have a higher risk factor for life-threatening diseases. In men especially, it's also an indicator of strength—the ability to protect and provide for their mate and offspring. So, judging a potential partner's body isn't entirely shallow. Just by assessing someone's looks, we can better determine their probability of being healthy in the longterm, and that same assessment greatly determines whether we want to sleep with them or not.

If you're married or you're in a relationship, this is obviously less of a concern for you. Even in a relationship, though, people want their spouse or partner to find them attractive. Relationships take work. If you think you went through all

**Even in a relationship, though, people want their spouse or partner to find them attractive. Relationships take work.**

that trouble to look good and put your best self out there and now that you've gotten a mate, your job is over, you're wrong. Let's be honest. If your partner isn't making an effort to look good anymore, it's easy for you to feel taken for granted. That's not to say the other person is at fault. A relationship is a two-way street, one that requires both partners to inspire each other, set new goals and challenges for themselves, and grow as individuals and as a couple. Fitness is going to bring all of those elements together to make a relationship stronger. The lasting attraction you have toward your mate is an expression of love, signifying that you want to be your best self for your partner. Fitness brings challenges, too. It takes the relationship to another level by engaging in activities that create a new lifestyle that will help you spend as many enjoyable and healthy years as possible together.

Many times, the spark in a relationship dies because people let themselves go and stop trying to embrace new challenges. Complacency sets in, and people begin to drift apart. But a lot of those things can be helped. We see it every day at BBB, where one partner joins, transforms her body in a very short time, and the other partner gets involved either after feeling the pressure to push himself or after just feeling inspired to get healthier when he sees his mate's progress. A couple comes in, works out together, and then finds a relationship revived and refocused.

Of all the life areas we'll get into, the visual element is the most obvious. I mention it here only to help you understand the larger impact even the most superficial component of fitness has on one's life.

## HEALTHY PARENTING

Now, as an extension of family and relationships, let's talk briefly about fitness's role in raising children. Physical activity is fairly routine among young kids. Their activities, education, and hobbies usually involve some type of physicality. But what happens as they get older? They could start spending more time playing video games or staring at their computers than they do being active. Perhaps they don't develop their eating habits and continue eating candy and junk food despite a slowing metabolism and a decline in physical activity. How kids develop good fitness habits comes down to your leadership. None of us should depend on athletes or celebrities to be the leaders for our children. If they are, it's because the parents have dropped the ball. As a parent, you may not be standing out as a leader to them, and a lot of that comes from the way in which you take care of yourself. If their parents are not in good health, kids tend to think they aren't the best examples to follow.

If you're involved in recreational drugs or you overuse alcohol, if you're overeating and not staying fit, then you're not blazing a healthy path for your children to follow. This is the first generation of children that is predicted to live fewer years than their parents, the first one in human history. That's 100 percent because of the obesity epidemic.[2] Your kids should want to be like you, so give them something to model themselves after that will make their lives healthier and more fulfilling.

## FINANCIAL FITNESS

Relationships and family life are going to be very dependent on fitness, but let's keep going. I mentioned earlier that fitness will impact your finances. I admit that it sounds hard to believe at first, but making money is also related to your personal fitness. How? It goes back to the primal aspect of fitness. Before there were tailored suits, push-up bras and Spanx, or the sign on your desk to let everyone know you're the boss, people knew who the leader was through that person's physical power. They knew who to follow from the impact such people made on those around them, mostly because of the way they carried themselves through their strength and energy. It wasn't necessarily the biggest person who was the leader of the pack, but rather the one who commanded the most respect. And a lot of that respect came from the confidence afforded by good physical appearance and capabilities.

---

2   Pam Belluck, "Children's Life Expectancy Being Cut Short by Obesity," *New York Times*, March 17, 2005, accessed September 3, 2017, http://www.nytimes.com/2005/03/17/health/childrens-life-expectancy-being-cut-short-by-obesity.html.

Today, when people look for leadership at work, for leadership at work, they're usually looking for leadership in general. Almost all of that comes back to how you're taking care of your body. People who take care of their bodies are usually in good health, and people in good health have a different energy about them. They seem like go-getters, ready for a challenge at all times.

The amount of hours you can put into your job will also be impacted by your fitness level. The quality of your sleep and the foods you eat, which are part of your fitness regimen, ultimately determine your energy and productivity throughout the day. If you prioritize your fitness, I can almost guarantee that you will be more successful in your work than you would be if you showed up on Mondays hung over or otherwise exhausted from a poorly spent weekend.

## BODY OVER MIND

We talked about the role fitness plays in your finances, relationships, and even your family, but let's get back to the most fundamental benefit of health and fitness. Feeling better about yourself is really what ties together all these areas of your life. Your mood, your confidence and energy levels, even the longevity of your life, are all directly related to your fitness.

Still, even in the face of this fact, we all make excuses. Some of us have more excuses or remain more defiant in dropping them than others, but we're all guilty of making excuses for our bad fitness choices. We look to examples of people who appear to have great lives without being in remotely good shape. Keith Richards, for instance, is a celebrity I hear people often cite as proof that poor fitness choices won't hurt you. Sure, you can say that Keith has had a lot of success in his career as a Rolling Stone and that despite his drug and alcohol use, his smoking, and whatever else, he's still going. But how might his life have been impacted had he been in better shape, had he spent his time making better choices for his body and mind instead of enduring all those years of abuse?

**Image and stamina are keys to success in the entertainment business.**

In the world of entertainment, we see the many positive effects of improving one's fitness. Image and stamina are keys to success in the entertainment business. Take as an example one of the hottest actors in Hollywood right now, Chris Pratt. In the span of just two years, Pratt went from relative anonymity to the star of such blockbusters as the *Guardians of the Galaxy* series, *Jurassic World*, *The Magnificent Seven*, *The Lego Movie*, and *Passengers*. Chris had been an actor for many years before landing those roles, having spent six years on the hit television show *Parks & Recreation* and playing small roles in several movies, but he was a sideline actor. He had confidence, a good sense of humor, and was succeeding in a demanding and competitive career. But by changing his body, making himself a model of fitness, Chris turned himself into the hottest actor in Hollywood. It goes to show what kind of impact your fitness level has.

You would think that if it were a perfect world, his improvement in his acting career would be related to taking a Shakespeare course or getting better at acting or landing a good role, but no, he changed his look and it changed his life.

Whether inspired by a celebrity like Chris, friends, a loved one, a personal health scare, or just by taking note of the cultural shift occurring around them, people are finally making comprehensive personal fitness mainstream. Nothing pumps me up more than seeing others realize their power to completely change their life and forge the future they want for themselves just by getting in shape.

This is a relatively new phenomenon. Our parents and grandparents weren't even aware that people could change their mind, spirit, and overall physical health so drastically just by changing their body. And that's what it's all about, really. When it comes to confidence and feeling comfortable in your own skin, it goes back to your body. If you start the day by jumping in the shower or changing your clothes and you're not happy with the first thing you see in the mirror, you're starting the day feeling like a failure.

> **Our parents and grandparents weren't even aware that people could change their mind, spirit, and overall physical health so drastically just by changing their body.**

To avoid that moment, you hurry to throw your clothes on or just skip looking in the mirror altogether. So, you're going to lack confidence in everything you do because you'll always feel something is missing. In some way, you feel incomplete, and unless you do something about it, you always will. Perhaps that's why you're holding this book. If it is, congratulations. You have made a huge and tremendously difficult first step by admitting that something is wrong and deciding to make a change to fill that void in your life and uncover the real you, the better version of yourself that you've always wanted to be.

Lastly—and it almost goes without saying—fitness is the best defense against disease. Period. Whether it's cancer, diabetes, heart disease, ailments of the joints, back problems, organ function, stroke, high cholesterol, high blood pressure—almost every common disease out there has a root cause stemming from your fitness level. It plays a role like no other in determining whether the time you have on earth is spent feeling healthy and energetic or feeling tired and cranky, going in and out of the hospital.

**Lastly—and it almost goes without saying—fitness is the best defense against disease. Period.**

Your fitness plays a major role in determining how much time you're going to have on planet Earth, and to what degree you'll enjoy that time, too. Again, a lot of it is genetics. If your parents or grand-parents lived to a ripe old age, then you may be starting with an advantage. If they did not, or if there are diseases commonly found in your family history, then you're going to have to step up and do something about it for your longevity.

The quality of your life while you're alive defines whether you're alive at all. Will you take on new experiences and adventures, spending time outdoors, traveling, meeting new and exciting people, and experiencing happy times? Or will you give in to doing the same old thing on the couch every night or hanging out with the same uninspiring people? Will you *choose* to lack confidence and hide in the shadows, or will you choose to step out into the light and lead the pack? If you ask me, I believe the quality of your life will be determined by your commitment to personal fitness. There just isn't a more important area of life.

★ ★ ★ ★ ★ ★ ★ ★ ★ ★ ★ ★ ★ ★ ★ ★ ★ ★ ★ ★ ★ ★ ★ ★ ★ ★ ★ ★ ★ ★ ★ ★

# CHAPTER 1 BBB QUESTIONNAIRE

Write a few sentences on how improving your fitness level will improve each of the following areas of your life:

### YOUR INTIMATE RELATIONSHIP:

*How will a better body add a spark? How much more will you be able to bring to the table?*

### YOUR FAMILY LIFE:

*Will your stress levels improve? In what ways will you be a better role model?*

### YOUR CAREER:

*Will greater energy and assertiveness pay off? Will you have more influence and be a better leader?*

### SPIRITUALITY:

*Will your body be a better temple? Will you have a higher sense of self-worth and self-discipline?*

### YOUR FRIENDSHIPS:

*Will you have higher value socially? Will you be a more fun person to be around?*

### YOUR LEISURE ACTIVITIES:

*What new and different fitness activities will you be able to take on? Will you be able to do more outdoors?*

★ ★ ★ ★ ★ ★ ★ ★ ★ ★ ★ ★ ★ ★ ★ ★ ★ ★ ★ ★ ★ ★ ★ ★ ★ ★ ★ ★ ★ ★ ★

# CHAPTER 2

# A BROKEN SYSTEM

People's fitness struggles today have less to do with the individual than they do with everything that surrounds that individual. We can't be too hard on ourselves given the amount of things wrong with the present state of fitness in our society. Virtually everything about the American lifestyle is set up against your personal fitness. Long workweeks that leave you with little time to spare, sedentary jobs, a fast food culture, rising expenses, and poor fitness instruction and education create a perfect storm for a very unhealthy lifestyle. Everything feels

> **Virtually everything about the American lifestyle is set up against your personal fitness.**

as if it's completely stacked against you, and I understand how over-whelming that feels when taken all at once. So, instead, let's look into each of those fitness obstacles a little more closely and figure out exactly what's happening.

★★★

**In the pages ahead, I'll show you the ideas behind building a Better Body by discussing:**

★ **The Broken Lifestyle**

★ **The Bad Food**

★ **The Other Drug Problem**

★ **The Coaching and Equipment Gap**

★ **The Environment and Experience Gap**

## THE BROKEN LIFESTYLE

I travel quite extensively to different parts of America and overseas. What I've found is that life in most developed countries today is designed to make you overweight, to make you live a less healthy life, and to grow more dependent on the medical community for help. It's not some grand conspiracy, I don't believe. It's just how a number of advancements in society have affected our general life-styles and diminished our fitness levels in the process, either directly or indirectly.

In the agricultural age, virtually everyone worked on a farm doing hard manual labor for several hours a day. In the industrial age, people still had to use their bodies. People still had to walk to wherever they worked. Most household activities involved manual labor as well. We're in the information age now when most jobs—even my job as a trainer and the head of a training business—require sitting. There couldn't be a worse thing for you. There's plenty of research out there showing how sitting shortens your life.[3] It's almost

---

3    Bonnie Berkowitz and Patterson Clark, "The Health Hazards of Sitting," *The Washington Post*, Jan. 20, 2014, accessed September 3, 2017, https://www.washingtonpost.com/apps/g/page/national/the-health-hazards-of-sitting/750/.

as bad as cigarettes, because your heart rate is so low for such an extended time.

When you're sitting, almost nothing is moving. Also, while chairs might have been invented for the sake of comfort, they're actually a very bad way to sit. They decrease your flexibility, impair your cardiovascular health, and reduce your muscle strength. To make matters worse, as soon as you leave work, you jump in the car and sit, only to get home and sit in front of the TV until you lie down in bed for the night. It becomes a habitual cycle that's terrible for your body.


## THE BAD FOOD

When you're driving home or sitting in front of that TV, you're inundated with messages about food. The problem is, almost every kind of food that's thrown at you in commercials is, to some degree, genetically engineered to make you fat. The ingredients in fast food are engineered with specific proportions of fat, starch, salt, and other preservatives and chemicals that make you crave more, whether you're hungry or not. Foods high in starches, fat, sugars, and preservatives can trigger an irregular insulin response. The more you eat, the more you have to eat in order to feel full, because your insulin level has shot up so high.[4] This type of food has properties and characteristics that you will never find in any natural foods humans have eaten throughout their existence on earth. Foods that are almost entirely synthetic should serve as all the warning one needs to approach them with caution.

---

4    David Ludwig, "Dr. David Ludwig Clears Up Carbohydrate Confusion," The Nutrition Source, Harvard T. H. Chan School of Public Health, accessed September 3, 2017, https://www.hsph.harvard.edu/nutritionsource/2015/12/16/dr-david-ludwig-clears-up-carbohydrate-confusion/.

Now think of the ways these companies market the food to you. They have made an American lifestyle around the consumption of food. Hot cakes, pancakes, muffins—these very starchy foods are considered to be breakfast foods, and they are going to give you a bad start to your day. Then, you see mass consumption of chemical-laden drinks to overcome the drop in blood sugar because of the overly starchy breakfast. Give yourself a 5-Hour Energy or a Red Bull to keep your energy level up? No. You're better off being tired.

**Give yourself a Five Hour Energy or a Red Bull to keep your energy level up? No. You're better off being tired.**

Lunch these days isn't much better. At work you might sometimes be encouraged to skip lunch or grab something quick such as a sandwich, something else with a lot of starch, or settle for other foods such as a pizza or a hamburger, both of which have excessive fat and carb content.

Dinner foods are typically even higher in starch, such as pastas and casseroles. That was fine in the agricultural and industrial ages, when people were usually on their feet all day and tended to eat less. They could refill their glycogen levels (how your body stores carbohydrates) at the end of the day and get a good night's sleep. But the average American today consumes starchy carbs all day long while sitting for hours upon hours. That means any extra carbs consumed at dinner will turn into excess fat.

To make matters worse, dinner isn't over with the main course. Next comes ice cream, chocolate, baked goods, and other desserts. We're taught that such foods can be "comfort" or "cheat foods." After a hard workout or a bad day at work, you might hear a little voice telling you, "It's been a long day; you deserve a treat." The problem is, these foods are usually made with sugar and fat that our bodies have no idea how to process. Learning about ingredients and how they interact with your body is critical to your overall fitness success. You wouldn't put absurd amounts of sugar, fat, and salt into your car's gas tank and expect it to run well, so why put things into your body without knowing what they are and how they'll affect your performance?

When you look at lifestyle and cultural norms, such as watching the big game with a beer and a bag of chips, or going out somewhere and eating ice cream or cotton candy, it's no surprise that obesity is a nationwide epidemic. Bad food has pervaded every part of our day, offering a quick, cheap, and accessible break from our busy and stressful lives. Everyone wants to be at least a little fitter, but without a consistent and intense workout regimen, even one bad meal a day will really put you behind the eight ball in terms of your fitness. Resisting the barrage of bad foods around us takes a lot of willpower, work, and education to overcome.

**When you look at lifestyle and cultural norms, such as watching the big game with a beer and a bag of chips or going out somewhere and eating ice cream or cotton candy, it's no surprise that obesity is a nationwide epidemic.**

We're going to talk about all of this in more detail in Section III of the book, and I promise that you don't have to be a saint to eat healthy food. You can eat the foods you love to eat, even the "bad" ones, but I'll teach you how to eat them at times that don't take you off track. Even more importantly, you'll learn to make better choices and how to use your body to work with the foods you love instead of against them. Knowledge is the first piece of any new endeavor. The BBB approach is going to arm you with that knowledge. We're going to talk about how easy it is to adopt a lifestyle that allows you to make easy improvements to your activity level and the foods you use to replenish your body.

## THE OTHER DRUG PROBLEM

Another problem in the fitness system I encounter time and time again is people putting too much faith in the health care industry. People are living longer, so everyone seems to assume they're living better. That couldn't be further from the truth.

> **People are living longer, so everyone seems to assume they're living better. That couldn't be further from the truth.**

Pharmaceutical companies and medical professionals may offer pills and surgeries to bandage you up when you're broken, but if the root cause of the problem hasn't been addressed, then you'll be back on the operating table or back at the pharmacy over and over again. The medications are just artificially manipulating different parts of your body—your chemicals, your cholesterol level, your blood pressure, and so on—to think everything is fine when it's not. Cholesterol levels are tied completely to eating habits and activity level, but rather than making a change to their lifestyle, people ingest chemicals or submit to invasive surgeries.

The medical industry has gotten very adept at masking the problems. Rather than encouraging you to adopt a healthier lifestyle, doctors can just change an artery or implant an artificial device to keep your body running a little longer. There is little to no talk of preventive care, which is exactly what the fitness industry is about. Surgeons can completely clear a blocked passageway, but identifying that problem earlier and making appropriate lifestyle changes would have been much safer, more effective, and cheaper. "You can't breathe? Here's an inhaler for you. Your heart is not working well? Here's a pill for you. You want to lose weight? We have a surgery for that." All of these solutions just enable the vicious cycle to continue unless you change your lifestyle. Sure, lifestyle changes don't seem to be simple, but that's a misperception. When compared to the trauma of a lifetime of relying on pills, hospital visits, and going under the knife, they're by far the simplest option available.

Don't feel overwhelmed. Changing your lifestyle is actually much, much easier than you might think. Now, I know that's the tagline on every single fitness book out there, but I'm in this business. I've done the field work and am still getting my hands dirty every day. I promise you that after as little as two or three days of doing the right type of training and eating correctly, you'll see improvements in how you feel, move, and look. Just by using the tools discussed throughout this book, you're going to see tremendous changes in your overall well-being.

**Changing your lifestyle is actually much, much easier than you would think . . . After as little as two or three days of doing the right type of training and eating correctly, you'll see improvements in how you feel, move, and look.**

The body improvement cycle is addictive. By getting in better shape and feeling good about the results, you're going to want to go back to the gym for more. I've been talking about bad addictions, but this is a good addiction: addiction to self-improvement, to your natural energy, to the way you feel, and to a positive environment.

## THE COACHING AND EQUIPMENT GAP

Finding quality coaching is another major challenge in your fitness journey, and everyone else's too. Cultivating the fitness addiction safely and with the best results requires some professional coaching. When we think about other important things in life that we need help with, there are usually plenty of instructors and resources available. We're in a capitalistic society. If there's a need, you'll usually find that there are companies, programs, and professionals addressing that need very well. However, the one area where you don't find that kind of help is fitness. In fact, if you're looking for coaching to help you improve your life through fitness, you won't be able to find much quality help at all.

**Our standards for hiring and training at BBB are the most rigorous in the entire fitness industry.**

Sure, there are thousands of personal trainers out there, but more often than not, they themselves are poorly trained and lack the right kind of motivation. Our standards for hiring and training at BBB are the most rigorous in the entire fitness industry. Perhaps not surprisingly to those of you who have gone to a large gym in the past, the fitness industry does not look anything like what I've discussed so far. It's one of the biggest ironies you will find. The need for fitness coaching is higher than ever, and yet there are very few legitimate professionals to turn to for help.

Most people's first reaction to their fitness problem is to join a gym, and once they do, they find a huge place, a warehouse more or less, full of equipment they don't know how to use. Most of it is bodybuilding equipment with a few cardiovascular machines here and there. There's really nothing you can do with that equipment that's going to cater to the type of lifestyle and body we've talked about thus far. Training to be a bodybuilder is completely different from working out to be a healthier, fitter person, and the equipment and training styles at this type of gym prove it.

Weightlifting equipment is good for strength training, but unless you have a balanced routine, that one piece of equipment is not something you can use for half an hour and develop a functional, balanced body. Every one of those machines is designed to isolate. The effectiveness of the machine, by definition, is how much it can work one small section of the body without incorporating the rest. That's a useless type of strength to have in the real world. It just does not apply to building a better body.

Your body doesn't use one muscle or muscle group at a time in the real world, so why would you train that way? Bodybuilders work to isolate muscles. In other words, they want to make one part of their body, one muscle at a time, as big as possible. Your average gym best serves bodybuilders. Everyone else will find it, for the most part, useless. If you're a woman reading this book who's looking for a lean, toned, and able-looking body, something that turns heads, something that feels good and looks good no matter which way you turn, how could those gym machines get you the form you seek? If you're a man who needs to shed some pounds, getting big isn't your issue. Perhaps you want a little more size around your shoulders or in your forearms, but what you really want is visible muscles. Body-building machines will just hide some muscle under the fat. On top of that, they can't build a body with the agility, functionality, and strength that the methods I'm talking about can achieve. Balanced workouts that engage as many muscle groups and systems as possible simultaneously are how you get there.

That's what the cardio machines are for, right? Not exactly. Those machines are meant for extended periods of training at a moderate pace and on a single plane of movement. When you're running on a treadmill, for instance, you're just going straight ahead and doing nothing laterally. You'll get a better calorie burn than sitting on your couch, but not much more than that. Unless you're using a competent trainer or are already knowledgeable, a gym for most people is either a waste of time and money or a place to incur injuries that leave you never wanting to go to a gym again.

## THE ENVIRONMENT AND EXPERIENCE GAP

A key ingredient in developing better fitness habits is finding the right environment. The typical gym model is built around signing up as many people as possible. That means anybody and everybody is sought out and lured into joining the neighborhood gym. That sounds like a good idea, but it actually creates a very anonymous and impersonal environment, making people feel even more judged as a result. You'll see a few people in shape who are really sweating, but all the others are just kind of staring into space because they're unsure of what to do and how. You may see a woman who is in shape and a man going over to hit on her. It's not surprising that gyms have developed a reputation for not feeling comfortable or welcoming, especially for women.

You may have also found that many gyms cater to people without many responsibilities in life such as young singles who don't have a demanding career and a family to contend with, or retirees with plenty of time on their hands. But people who have a full, busy life with a lot of responsibilities are not going to feel comfortable in a gym like that, and a bad gym experience is one of the main reasons people get turned off fitness before the progress even begins.

> **A bad gym experience is one of the main reasons people get turned off fitness before the progress even begins.**

Think of the locker room environment. It's usually dirty and full of people you've never met before and will probably never hang out with, and now, you're getting naked next to them. It literally and figuratively reeks of a place you don't want to go to. If this is the only choice you have, then it's understandable why you're not working out.

Let's talk about the staff a little more, because a bad staff is why most gyms don't work for most people. Much of the industry is a do-it-yourself type of thing. The people who become trainers in a gym are some of the most underqualified people. Why? For many reasons, really.

One reason is that they don't have a high-paying position. No parents are excited for their son or daughter to become a personal trainer at the local gym, which is very unfortunate, because fitness training is one of the most important and rewarding careers if it's done correctly. People are desperately in need of coaching. They're in need of guidance, of streamlining the process to keep themselves healthy, and the people they turn to are, more often than not, completely incapable of helping them. That's almost universal in this business.

It takes very little to become a trainer these days. Just a simple test will give you a certification. The standards have become more rigorous, so you have to study a little bit longer for the test, but really, it says nothing about your ability as a motivator, your ability as a leader, or your ability to encourage a positive lifestyle. Usually, personal trainers are just glorified salespeople walking you through the motions. It's better than nothing, but not significantly.

So, you have all these things working against you: the food culture, the health care industry, the job, the family, the general lifestyle of unhealthiness. And what do you do? You turn to a gym, the main solution you know of, only to find that it's ultimately working against you. Your next knee-jerk reaction is to hire a trainer, only to find that's not an effective solution either. It's just a therapy session, a one-on-one, noncustomized routine led by an underqualified person.

That's the bad news, but don't let it get you down. I have good news for you too. Let's move on to see what's being done at BBB to combat these challenges and how you yourself can use them right now, wherever you are.

★ ★ ★ ★ ★ ★ ★ ★ ★ ★ ★ ★ ★ ★ ★ ★ ★ ★ ★ ★ ★ ★ ★ ★ ★ ★ ★ ★ ★ ★ ★

# CHAPTER 2 BBB QUESTIONNAIRE

Which of the following negative influences below are tripping you up?
Write a few sentences explaining, and describe the solutions:

## FAST FOOD:

*Are you making poor food choices out of convenience? How can you solve this?*

## SITTING:

*Are their periods of the day when you're getting too little physical activity and movement? What can you do to make your work and leisure time more active?*

## JUNK FOOD ADVERTISING:

*Are bad snack foods getting in your way? What can you do to make better eating and snack choices?*

## GYMS:

*Why haven't gyms worked for you in the past? Was it a bad environment? Was no one around to help?*

★ ★ ★ ★ ★ ★ ★ ★ ★ ★ ★ ★ ★ ★ ★ ★ ★ ★ ★ ★ ★ ★ ★ ★ ★ ★ ★ ★ ★ ★ ★

# CHAPTER 3

# A BETTER BODY, A BETTER WAY

I'm not all doom and gloom. I promise. Despite the numerous obstacles that stand in our way between our day-to-day lives and our fitness goals, there is hope. A big trend is spreading throughout the fitness industry right now, a very positive trend that's designed to maneuver around the lifestyle constraints of the average person. It's called boutique fitness, and while I've been training clients in this style for more than a decade, you can certainly call my company, BBB, a part of this trend.

So what is it? All boutique fitness means is that instead of a big-box-store type of fitness experience—the cheap products, the generic programs, the uncaring staff, the impersonal atmosphere—you are getting a specialized fitness program with expert trainers capable of tailoring a program around your needs and goals. Just its very nature brings clients into contact with like-minded people who have similar goals and lifestyles. This sense of community is critical to keeping you invested in your fitness for the long term. We'll talk about that in greater detail later on in the book.

**All boutique fitness means is that instead of a big-box-store type of fitness experience—the cheap products, the generic programs, the uncaring staff, the impersonal atmosphere—you are getting a specialized fitness program with expert trainers capable of tailoring a program around your needs and goals.**

I'm sure you've already guessed by now that BBB is a bootcamp-style gym, but what does that mean exactly? Mostly it just means that we train as a team. If you want a high-level workout that offers reliability and expert guidance from attentive trainers, then BBB is for you. Fitness bootcamps are supposed to offer a calorie burn designed to make you look great, while also focusing on a balanced approach to building your body. Unfortunately, not all bootcamp-style programs are created equally.

Bootcamps were something I stumbled upon early on in my training career, but most of them were very expensive, very harsh, and short-term. People traveled from afar to attend a camp for a day, a weekend, or sometimes longer, but that was it. Then they all went home and were expected to have been so transformed that they would continue doing sit-ups in the mud for the rest of their life. These bootcamps just didn't work for me, so I decided to look for something different, something better.

I started training clients professionally a little more than fifteen years ago, and what I found was an industry that was more obsessed with the mode than the results. Training programs have gotten better, smarter across the board in some ways, but as I've said before, most trainers and gyms are still significantly lacking in quality and effectiveness.

I wanted to offer something more to my clients, something that really worked, so they would keep their commitment to fitness for

**"I'm sure you've already guessed by now that Better Body Bootcamp is a bootcamp-style gym, but what does that mean exactly? Mostly it just means that we train as a team... a high-level workout that offers reliability and expert guidance from attentive trainers."**

longer and really be able to reap the benefits of being healthy. So, I started BBB in 2011 with that mission in mind. From the beginning, my team and I designed our gym around clients who seek a functional approach to fitness. We want to ensure that everything about the body we're creating for our clients looks good, feels good, and functions well together. You want a balanced body. You want to be able. You want to be limber. You want to be strong. You want to look

**From the beginning, my team and I designed our gym around clients who seek a functional approach to fitness. We want to ensure that everything about the body we're creating for our clients looks good, feels good, and functions well together.**

and feel great. And you want to do it in the least amount of time possible. That's what everyone wants. How we get there is almost irrelevant. **It has to be positive. It has to be effective. It has to be safe.** That's the code we live by at BBB.

We also approach training differently. How? Well, in a technical nutshell, we like things such as cross training, muscle confusion, interval training, and body-part-specific conditioning to achieve a lean, toned, defined, and able body. In good gyms, for instance, you'll find a kettlebell class. The purpose of kettlebell training is to work the whole body, but these classes are limiting themselves by using this piece of equipment alone. Kettlebell training is a huge part of what we do here at BBB too, but it's not the only tool we use in any given class. We use it in conjunction with other techniques and tools, enabling you to keep pushing and diversifying your training with every class. Spin classes are another major fad right now, but again, it's only one type of equipment working one area of your body (cardiovascular) in one type of way. Where's the strength aspect? Kickboxing is another trend, and it's great. We're big believers in it here too, so we incorporate it into our interval training program. But again, if kickboxing is the only thing you do, you're only getting a cardiovascular workout from your class. At a certain point, your body is going to get used to it, and you're going to stop getting results.

BBB is about taking your body to its best form through incremental levels. It's a new evolution in training by being a result-centered program that chooses from all types of fitness routines, training techniques, and nutrient-processing responses to build a body specific to your design. We use all the tools I just mentioned (cardiovascular training, kettlebells, kickboxing, weight training) and more, but we use them in combination, rotating them in and out according to how your body responds. We don't let the tools limit us. We use the proper tool for the job at hand. You use a hammer to drive in a nail, a screwdriver for a screw. We're using whatever it takes to get you looking your absolute best, and the most scientifically proven techniques are part of what we do here.

Intervals are important. That's a big part of what we do. Core strength? Yes, we do it. Functional training? Yes, we do that too. Then there are some benefits to a physique-training approach. In fact, body-part-specific training is a big component of what happens here. Many of those same ideas are what you're going to learn about later in this book.

**It's a new evolution in training by being a result-centered program that chooses from all types of fitness routines, training techniques, and nutrient-processing responses to build a body specific to your design.**

This book will set up the game, so to speak. It will teach you the rules, show you the tools and tricks, and educate you on how to approach *your* body, building the body you want in the best way possible. My mission is to make working out a natural part of your life, and I'll do that by showing you how to start making a positive long-term change in your lifestyle by seeing and feeling the results right away.

## THE ORIGINS OF BBB

When I got into fitness, it was for the same reasons many young men get into it: to be bigger and stronger than my peers. I was twelve or thirteen when I first started lifting weights. For me, I wanted to grow up a lot faster, to be a man already. By the time I was in high school, I was the fittest of any of my friends and one of the strongest and fittest in my grade. I loved the power, for lack of a better word, that being fit gave me.

Rather than being the bully, I was actually the other kids' protector from the bullies. I gained a lot of great friends because of it, and in a way, I find it to be my role as a trainer as well. In terms of fitness and health, it seems everything is coming after people these days. Because I was predisposed to fitness early on, I feel I'm the one standing up for them, in a different way, using fitness to help people fight back.

We have trainers on our staff who were once very overweight. They're now in much better shape than I am, and their physical transformation makes them people our clients can relate to or be inspired by. They've actually created a lifestyle change, and it's working out tremendously well for them.

I'm one of those people who came out of the womb wanting to be very fit and physically in shape, so I started doing something about it sooner than most. But my passion for training didn't begin until I entered college.

Remember the medical and pharmaceutical industries we talked about in the last chapter? I'm more familiar with them than most. My road to a career in medicine started with a five-year undergraduate degree course in pharmacy.

During my first few years in college, I was an A student on the Dean's List. I loved my studies, both the liberal arts or sciences. But when the studies began focusing more on drugs and chemicals, I hated them. I became disillusioned with the field as it seemed to be more about passing out pills than solving problems and preventing the need for drugs in the first place. I took enough classes in pharmacology to figure out how much you can manipulate the chemicals in your body with these drugs and how easily you can completely mask, not cure, the negative effects of your lifestyle. I'm not denigrating pharmacists. I know many of them and think they're great people doing good work, but even they nod their head in agreement with me over problems in the industry related to preventive care.

Eventually, I decided to change my course of studies to biology to learn more about what truly fascinated me: the human body. I wanted to understand how the body works and how it interacts with external factors. By the time I finished my college education, I wanted to be a trainer. I immediately got my certification and started training at a local gym, which was a shocking experience. It was like being a used car salesman. Trainers hovered around the sales floor, trying to pick up a client. Many of them had zero education. In fact, there was no mention of education at all when it came to personal training.

Nonetheless, being in the gym and working with my first few clients made me more determined than ever. My clients came from all occupations, backgrounds, and levels of fitness experience. One client was a young, beautiful woman with a lot of drive, but at more than two hundred pounds, she needed to lose weight, and she needed to do it fast. Within a few weeks, I helped her lose her first ten pounds, and she never looked back. I watched her life transform as the pounds dropped. Her confidence and energy level climbed to new heights, and I was hooked. Another client, a woman in her fifties, had just had a pacemaker put in. Together, we drastically changed her eating and exercise habits and breathed new life into her. I trained many more clients who were just trying to look good on the beach, but regardless of their reasons, seeing people discover their best selves and create new lives was unbelievably satisfying.

After a few years, I decided to set out on my own. I had a good technical background already, but I made it my point to keep learning.

I went to all the seminars, read all the top books, and traveled around the country to meet as many top trainers as I could. I watched them train celebrities and professional athletes in state-of-the-art facilities. As a result, I've witnessed the genesis of just about every fitness trend and gadget popular today. I trained with the leaders of some of today's highly popular programs before they became popular and witnessed the emergence of kettlebells, and I remember when spinning was just, well, spinning.

I made it my mission to change the industry, to help trainers get out of big-box gyms and venture out on their own. I learned from the best in the business, such as Jake "Body by Jake" Steinfeld and Tony Horton from P90X. I really made it a point to learn from the best and find out how they were getting results.

So, how do they do it? They all focus on one area. Gunnar Peterson, for instance, only works with celebrities to get them in shape for their next movie. Todd Durkin is focused on getting someone to run faster or be more powerful. Tony Horton's P90X is a great program that adopts many theories and techniques from muscle confusion and focuses on excess weight loss.

For most people, though, these programs and specialties are not appropriate. People who have failed to get themselves in shape because of time or lifestyle obstacles certainly won't benefit from Gunnar's techniques or Todd's style of training. There are only a few out there for whom weight gain is not an issue, possibly because they are genetically or metabolically fortunate in some way.

We have a wide array of members at BBB, and because we customize members' plans, they're able to be appropriately challenged in an environment that's inclusive regardless of their skills or experience level. Some are former athletes who are trying to reclaim their fitness now that their playing days are gone. Many more are just regular folks with families and careers, some who have never played a sport or been physically active. We make a regimen that challenges everyone equally by creating a program that's proportional to an individual's abilities.

## THE BBB WAY

I told you at the beginning of this book that fitness is the most important part of life. You can pick up any book or turn on any TV channel focused on fitness and you won't find fitness viewed in that way. But all of my clients know it. If they

**We have a wide array of members at BBB, and because we customize members' plans, they're able to be appropriately challenged in an environment that's inclusive regardless of their skills or experience level.**

didn't know it before they came to me, they certainly know it by the time they leave. They're almost staking their life on it. That's why, at BBB, we treat your fitness as a matter of life and death. We don't leave anything to chance.

In most of today's gyms, trainers are regarded as little more than order-takers instead of being in a position to change, or even save, lives. The average person sees going to a gym as something of an act of leisure. Making a change is voluntary, and that's why you have to be the leader in how you approach your eating and your fitness. But good trainers are leaders. They're there to inspire you, to keep you motivated through the pain and discouraging times. All of our trainers here at BBB are professionals who also serve as leaders in our community because we treat the business the way it should be treated.

When fitness is done correctly, it benefits the whole community by improving individual lives while bringing people together. At BBB, we organize events year-round that inspire people to challenge themselves and reach for something greater. When our clients learn they're capable of exceeding their own expectations in the gym, they never want to stop exploring their limits, whether it be in fitness or any other area of their life.

Interestingly, even though social media has put more people in touch with one another, people have simultaneously grown more and more isolated. That's one reason I wanted BBB to be a place where people could work toward common goals together and be in physical contact with like-minded people every single day. People crave meaningful connection now more than ever. Whether you agree with your workout partner's opinions on Facebook or not doesn't matter. When you're sweating and grinding through the pain together to create something better for your life, none of that makes any difference. In that moment, you're in it together.

We have accomplished something incredibly unique with our approach to fitness. I wouldn't be motivated to write this book, or to grow our program, if it weren't something special. We wouldn't have seen our success as one of the top, privately owned fitness companies in the country, either. With so many new members joining our movement daily, we've become the go-to fitness option in our local communities. It would be impossible to spur such a response if our program didn't work.

I honestly don't know where I got my interests and skills in fitness training. A lot of it was hard work. And I was born with some of it. It's certainly been a path with a lot of twists and turns, but with a little luck and a lot of great people getting behind us at BBB, we have created what can only be described as a revolution in the way people think about fitness.

What I do know is that we have done it all with one goal in mind: the never-ending quest to find the ideal mode of training. Every decision is made based on how we can create a more time-efficient and body-effective program, regardless of a person's fitness level, one that surpasses every other fitness program available. I've spent my career trying to solve that problem, and while I'm obviously biased, I believe BBB has found the best solution to the general public's fitness challenges in a way that no other program in the country has. It starts by learning about who you are, where your fitness level is, where you want it to be, and what you need in order to get there. The change begins with a simple question: Why are *you* here?

★ ★ ★ ★ ★ ★ ★ ★ ★ ★ ★ ★ ★ ★ ★ ★ ★ ★ ★ ★ ★ ★ ★ ★ ★ ★ ★ ★ ★ ★ ★ ★ ★ ★ ★ ★

# CHAPTER 3 BBB QUESTIONNAIRE

The Better Body approach makes the absolute most out of your specific genetic gifts and strengths while eliminating your weaknesses. Describe how this relates to you personally below:

### WHAT YOU LOVE:

*What are the best parts of your body? What are your genetic strengths?*

### THINGS TO IMPROVE:

*What are your weaknesses? What are the areas you want to improve?*

### YOUR BODY TYPE:

*Do you have a generally skinny body type, or more shapely or stocky? Who are some celebrities or people in the media that are making the most out of your body type?*

### YOUR PREDISPOSITIONS:

*What type of fitness activities do you love? How can you enjoy them more?*

### YOUR GOALS:

*What are your specific body goals? What are your eating goals?*

★ ★ ★ ★ ★ ★ ★ ★ ★ ★ ★ ★ ★ ★ ★ ★ ★ ★ ★ ★ ★ ★ ★ ★ ★ ★ ★ ★ ★ ★ ★ ★ ★ ★

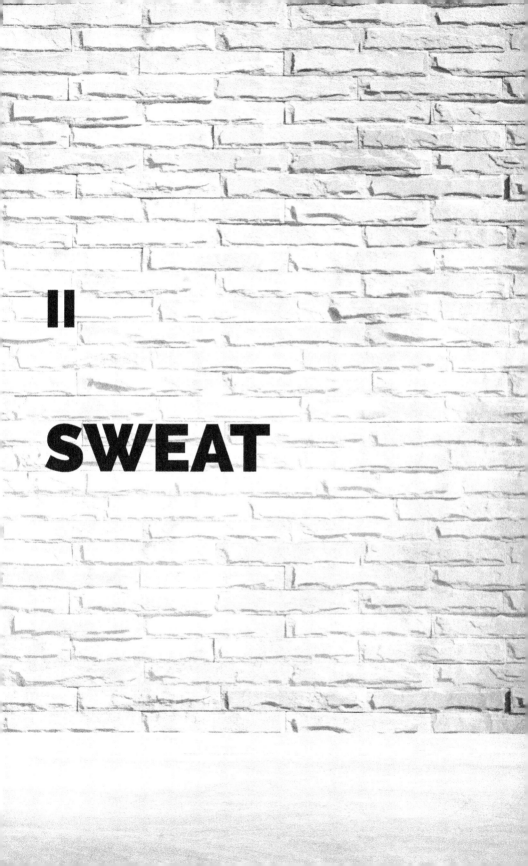

# II

# SWEAT

# CHAPTER 4

# HOW TO TRAIN

**N**ow that you know why fitness is so important and what your personal goals are, let's talk about changing your body. What are the steps and techniques for transforming the body at BBB? As we discussed in Chapter 3, BBB bases its fitness approach on the most effective ways to train, incorporating the same research and methods from the top experts in the industry into each of our customized programs.

Obviously, I can't review your answers to the BBB Questionnaires in previous chapters as I would in a one-on-one consultation, but I imagine you have some concerns related to aesthetics, simply because we all do. How we look in the mirror and feel about our body is perhaps the most popular reason for coming to us. You may want to have your problem zones tightened up or shrunk, or add muscle to certain parts of your body. Or perhaps you love your shape and size and just want to maintain it. All of that and more can be achieved with this system.

BBB's training program is built around a set of principles we call the **better body breakthroughs**. Some of the points below may be new to you, because, after all, if everyone knew them, more people would have an easier time getting in shape. Many of these points may be things you've already heard or are already doing. That's okay too. BBB is the only program that incorporates them all, and that's the real breakthrough we're talking about here.

> **BBB's training program is built around a set of principles we call the better body breakthroughs.**

How to combine them into a fitness program that's "fool-proof" is what I will show you how to do in this book.

★ **BREAKTHROUGH #1: Your training must be body-part specific.** Strength training needs to have a purpose. You *can* have the body aesthetic you want in addition to good overall fitness.

★ **BREAKTHROUGH #2: Your training must be functional.** Why work one muscle group when you can work many? While you're developing a tighter, more toned chest, why not work your core too? When working your arms and shoulders, why not incorporate your legs and butt at the same time? Cutting down your overall training time while greatly improving your results is a no-brainer.

★ **BREAKTHROUGH #3: You have to keep your body guessing.** Does your gym routine look pretty much the same every time you go? You can create muscle confusion to drive and extend your goals. As soon as your body figures out what you're doing, it stops adapting and you stop seeing the fruits of your labor. You must challenge your body to continue getting results. If your heart rate isn't accelerated, if you're not sweating and breathing hard, then you need to increase your pace, weight, repetitions, and so on, until you are.

★ **BREAKTHROUGH #4: You have to train in groups.** Gyms, and even personal trainers, often make training a solo activity. It takes a village to get your body into the best possible shape.

★ **BREAKTHROUGH #5: Your training has to be fun.** Forget about grueling New Year's resolutions. Putting your workout as yet another item on your to-do list is the best way to sabotage your success. Exercise can't be a chore. If it is, it will be the first thing you ditch when your schedule gets busy. It has to be the highlight of your day.

★ **BREAKTHROUGH #6: Your training must be comprehensive.** Specialized boutique fitness programs usually fail before they even get started because they restrict themselves to only one type of training or movement. Your training regimen must be multidimensional, include cardio intervals, targeted weight training, functional training, flexibility, and core-strengthening movements. Just taking a spin class may get you lean, but it won't get you toned.

Your regimen has to have it all, in a smart and balanced combination.

★ **BREAKTHROUGH #7: You have to exercise consistently.** Forget about being a weekend warrior or meeting your trainer twice a week. The body is meant to move every day. This is a lifelong pursuit. A program must be consistent, and it needs to challenge you physically every day. It's not something you'll be doing twelve hours a day, but it's something that needs attention, in some way, every single day.

★ **BREAKTHROUGH #8: Your training must have a purpose.** Without a challenging and meaningful goal, it's hard to stay motivated. You have to know what you're going after. Your goals must be clear, and you must revisit them often. If there's a dress, suit, or whatever that you want to look good in, keep that by your bedside and try it on every few days to see how you're doing. Another option is to plan a vacation somewhere hot, so you'll be forced to get yourself ready to look good in less clothing than usual.

★ **BREAKTHROUGH #9: Train safely.** If you're injured, you can't work out. Safety is paramount. Your workout regimen shouldn't be so painfully grueling that you cause more harm to your body than good.

★ **BREAKTHROUGH #10: Train with a professional.** With your busy life, you don't have the time to become an expert fitness coach for yourself. You need some level of coaching to reach your goals effectively and safely.

## THE TEN BETTER BODY BREAKTHROUGHS

Let's look at these breakthroughs in a little more detail, beginning with **appearance geared strength training** in your routine. What I mean by that is there needs to be some strength training, but strength training with a purpose. Now, some of the recent focus in the fitness industry has been on functional fitness. Traditional moves that improve your appearance have gone out of vogue. I've spoken to many gym owners who told me that body-part-targeted, aesthetic strength training is not what they do. They offer performance programs.

We talked about how the fitness industry is broken. Bodybuilding is, in a typical gym, not the way you'd want to train to get your best body. Maybe you want to lose a little weight—or on the opposite spectrum, gain general muscle—but are you going to be left with the body that you really wanted by using bodybuilding techniques? It's not likely. We can design a program that's going to get you functionally fit, burn fat, gain muscle, *and* get you the kind of body aesthetic you want. They're not mutually exclusive.

That same idea is why **functional training** is so important. When we're focusing on your legs, we need to keep the aesthetic in mind. We can't just go and start doing heavy-weighted squats. If you're a woman who's overweight, your legs will get bigger. But what if the point was to get your legs smaller? If your arms are big and we're trying to decrease the size of your arms, concentrating on the arms in a thoughtless way isn't going to help. We need to keep that in mind.

At the end of this chapter, you will find instructions for a few exercises of this type. Functional training is all we do at BBB. For example, the leg exercises we choose are meant to shape your butt, but they keep the size of your thighs in mind as well so they don't get too big. The abdominal exercises we choose to work with shrink your waist while toning your stomach. The upper-body exercises, for a woman, keep her looking lean but still toned and functional.

I imagine men are trying to "cut up" that upper body. For male readers of this book, size is probably not the problem. If you are trying to significantly bulk up, this isn't the system you should use. There are many other good books that address that workout style. But if you want to get lean and toned, this is the book for you. You'll find some of those exercises at the end of the chapter as well.

Our third and sixth breakthroughs go hand-in-hand as they're all about the need to have a body-part split system, or **muscle confusion**, and keeping the workout regimen comprehensive, meaning working out all the muscle groups evenly. We need to train different muscle groups on different days of the week to give you a lean, toned, and balanced body. What you're going to find these days is that a lot of the popular programs focus on full-body exercises every day. What that means is you're going to eventually outgrow them. Bootcamp training typically refers to an obstacle course where physical activity is designed to burn calories and make you sweat. This is great, but you're not going to get a comprehensive workout. You'll gain stamina. You'll gain strength. You'll get in good shape, but then you'll hit a plateau. If you did the exercise in the last section correctly, I hope you set some extremely ambitious goals. Plateauing is not part of the equation. We want to keep going. Targeting different muscle groups on different days of the week is one way we're going to achieve that.

Going back to the example of bodybuilding, people using that workout style have a leg day, an upper body day, a back day, a shoulder day, a butt day, and so on. There's a lot of value in that because you have to focus on each area of the body throughout the week. We use the same idea at BBB.

On leg day at BBB, for example, we're focusing on legs predominantly but not exclusively. Your legs are working very hard on those days, meaning you have a lot of blood moving to that area. We're going to work them from multiple angles, which is what you need to keep in mind for a balanced approach. When we're working just one area—for example, legs or arms—you want to hit every part of the arms or legs. We want to get every ounce out of that muscle. Another term I use is *wringing them out like a towel*: squeezing every bit out of a given muscle group and then letting it recover for the next few days.

Friday will be something like a full-body day. Your upper body is recovered because it was exercised earlier in the week, so we'll focus on it again and do some cardiovascular work that involves your legs. That's a full-body day. Then Saturday is a cardio-only day when we don't hit the weights hard. Instead, we just train your most important muscle: your heart.

That brings me to another key point we need to keep in mind: the importance of using functional equipment. Typical gym equipment is not going to do it for you. This is one of the hardest habits for people to break because, subconsciously, when you walk into a gym, you feel you have to use the equipment. Why would they have devoted the entire gym to this 1980s-era, single-joint/single-muscle-group type of equipment if that wasn't the best way to train?

As I said, it's a remnant of the 1980s, when bodybuilders who took drugs and steroids were genetically gifted, had radical diets, and looked good on magazine covers, but it's not the '80s anymore. That way of training is not going to get a busy person like you or me in shape, nor is the equipment going to be very helpful.

For example, my friend Gunnar Peterson has a gym full of every type of contraption known to man, and he needs it all because his clients are top athletes and movie stars, not everyday people.

> **It's not the '80s anymore. That way of training is not going to get a busy person like you or me in shape, nor is the equipment going to be very helpful.**

You'll also find that top trainers like Gunnar will modify gym equipment to target a specific body part and get the result they're looking for. We want to be body-part specific too, but we want to train functionally at the same time. Most traditional equipment simply can't do both.

In a gym, you would train your chest with a chest machine or with some dumbbells while lying on your back. Every other part of your body is at rest except the chest. But what if we replaced working out on a chest press with a decline pushup (your feet would be elevated)? Think of the subtle change in the many muscle groups that are now involved. Your core is engaged to a huge degree, along with your legs, triceps, biceps, shoulders, and of course, your chest.

We're talking about having a nice body, and you can't achieve that without adapting a comprehensive fitness program. Just as weightlifting alone won't get you "cut" or increase your stamina, running for several days in a row won't do anything for you strength-wise. That's the benefit of functional training: it allows you to attack the body from top to bottom at the same time.

If you have a BBB location close to you, you'll discover that's entirely the best way to train. We're trying to do several things at once with every exercise.

**Community** is another critical component of the BBB training strategy. As I mentioned in Chapter 1, exercising is one of the most primal things we do in today's world, so doing it as part of a "tribe" makes total sense. You need to be around people who support and inspire you. You need to be a leader for other people, and they need to be leaders for you when your motivation drops or you feel discouraged, as we all do from time to time.

That brings us to our next breakthrough: **it has to be fun**. That's the bottom line. In today's world, just finding an hour of quality time with your significant other or your kids can be tough. Now you have to find an hour most days of the week to get yourself in shape, so if it's seen as a chore, it'll be the last thing you do.

We have to find a way to make you look forward to working out. The right community is going to help tremendously, but the actual exercises and classes you take part in have to be fun, too. After all, there's only so much a great community can do to keep you engaged in a regimen that isn't fun.

Our goal is to make our program something that will inspire you to keep fighting through a rough day at work so you can come to the gym and get a release with friends. BBB is about feeling good, looking good, releasing stress, and finding community. If we can achieve that, we know it will be the highlight of your day.

The next breakthrough is that it must be **highly effective**. That might sound redundant because I've already spelled out many breakthroughs that will make your program effective, but it needs to be *highly* effective. It needs to be done at the correct intensity, and every breakthrough I've discussed has to be incorporated, or something major will be missing.

Some of the elements of an effective workout regimen are what we've talked about already: it must be body-part targeted and functional, maintain the right intensity, and be comprehensive. All of those elements are key to a successful regimen, but the bottom line is this: the greatest motivator for exercise is great results. Turning heads—or even doing double-takes at yourself—is one of the best things to help you stick with the program.

Our seventh breakthrough is **consistency**. To be successful, a workout regimen needs to be done every single day. The body is meant to move every day. Life before modern times was all about movement. Lo and behold, obesity was not a problem. Now, it's not about movement at all. You need to train in some way every single day to build an amazing body.

Consistency is one of the key things I picked up from a mentor of mine, Tony Horton. I trained with Tony several years ago, and one of the main reasons Tony's famed P90X program works so well is because it is an everyday program. I still talk with Tony regularly and continue to learn a lot from him, and he says one of the key reasons his program works is because it's designed to move the body every day. We took the same stance when developing BBB. It's not as if you have to come to BBB every day, or run or strength train every day, but you're going to have to do something effective every day.

Our next breakthrough is **purpose**. That was the point of the goals that we talked about in the last chapter. I had you write your goals, and I want you to keep those goals clear. You need to revisit them. I talked about how you need to have body role models: a celebrity that has a similar body type to yours, is of a similar age to you, and whose physique you admire. If you're a short guy in your fifties, for instance, your body role model could be Tom Cruise. If you're a tall guy who's feeling a little too skinny, you could use Chris Hemsworth or Idris Elba as a body model.

If you're a woman who's more curvy, Angelina Jolie (who doesn't have that type of body) won't work, but Alicia Keyes, Jennifer Lopez, Beyoncé, or someone of that build might. The bottom line is you need to have goals. You need to have a purpose. You have to know what you're working for.

One of my pet peeves with fitness programs is that they make working out a sport. Working out is not a sport; it is training to get something done. You want to lose an inch off your waist, there's a suit or dress you want to look good in again—that kind of want becomes your purpose. You need to be clear about your goals because they're going to motivate you when you get busy and the going gets rough.

**Safety** is our ninth breakthrough. A great program needs to be one that's safe, that won't injure you. A lot of the high-intensity, competition-based programs can cause injuries. I recently spoke to a physical therapist who said high-intensity and military-style bootcamps and races are the best things that ever happened to his business because of the huge number of injuries caused by those poorly supervised activities.

Safety is paramount at BBB. While many of our members range in age, from twenty to sixty, we know that most of our members are in their thirties and forties and aren't trying to break any high jump or bench-press records any time soon. All those in their thirties and forties will tell you that the body just doesn't move or react the way it used to. It needs to be safe.

The tenth and final breakthrough is to **train with a professional**. This may sound like an obvious plug, but whether you only work with a trainer to establish a regimen or work with one daily, consulting a trainer is very important to your success. A qualified trainer will help you determine your strengths and weaknesses, set goals, teach you the exercises and proper techniques needed to achieve them, and then hold you accountable. Without the help of a good trainer, you're putting your safety at risk as well as your chances of getting the body you want.

## CHAPTER 4 – BBB WORKOUT DEMO

Among the Better Body Breakthroughs is our revolutionary approach to strength training. It's an approach anyone interested in transforming their body can adopt. It doesn't matter where you are because it doesn't require a great deal of equipment to execute.

First, we choose exercises that specifically work to improve your appearance. Secondly, with the busy pace of life these days, these exercises must cram as much effort out of as many body parts as possible. This isn't functional training in the traditional sense. It's full-body training that gets the absolute most out of each body part worked.

In the following section, you'll find a few of the moves we do at Better Body, which, when put together, will constitute a full-body strength-training session that hits you from every angle. These movements were chosen because they will lend themselves toward creating a lean, toned, and balanced appearance.

One thing to keep in mind is that we mix each of these strength moves with high-intensity cardio intervals throughout our workouts. What that means is we rarely perform strength training in a sequence by itself. We always have cardio mixed into it in order to keep the heart rate high and the calories burned to the max.

Also, this represents just a tiny portion of the literally unlimited number of exercises you would find in a Better Body training session. Using the descriptions of each move, you'll learn some of the principles behind what we do and how we do it, and I hope you'll be able to create some diverse training regimens for yourself, too.

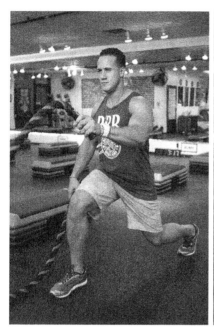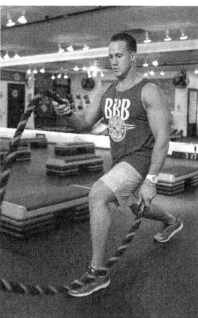

## 1. ALTERNATING LUNGE PLUS BATTLING ROPES
*(ARMS, LEGS, AND BUTT)*

Your arms are the most exposed part of your body, so it's important for them to look terrific. When working arms, we always like to mix legs in too, and that's why you see alternating reverse lunges combined with the battling ropes here. About the battling ropes: there's not a single other piece of equipment that's better for achieving amazing arms.

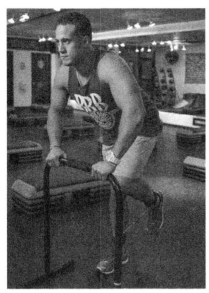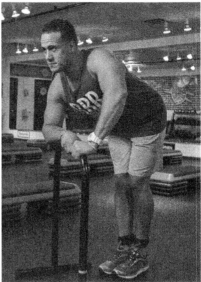

## 2. GLUTE SQUEEZE WITH BOOTY BANDS *(BUTT)*

Isolating your glutes serves two purposes. First, it's great focused, isolated work because they are among your marquee muscles. Secondly, this activates your glutes, meaning you learn to squeeze these muscles harder. This gives you added strength to all of your other leg exercises.

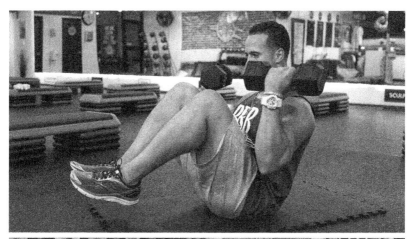

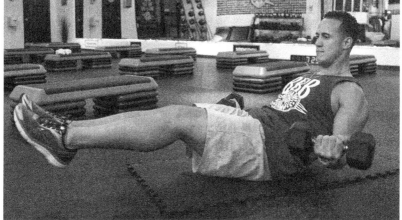

### 3. CURLS PLUS V-UP CRUNCH *(BICEPS AND ABS)*

When working arms, which are small muscle groups, we always like to get the rest of the body involved. That's what you find with the curls plus the v-up crunch. The biceps are the focus of the curls, with shoulders and chest also coming into play for stability. This curling motion is combined with a v-up crunch to also give intense attention to the abdominals.

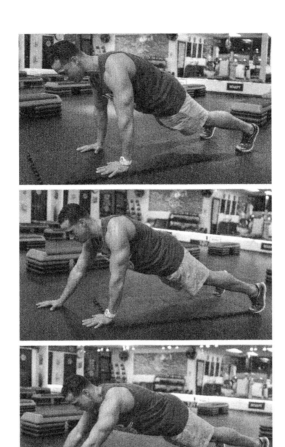

## 4. CRAWL OUTS *(BACK, ABS, AND LEGS)*

In my experience, no woman looking to get toned or a man trying to get lean is looking for a big, bulky back. That's why at Better Body, we always choose back exercises that are meant to tone, tighten, and define. Crawl outs are a favorite, not just because they hit your back, but because so many other major muscle groups come into play. The planking aspect of it will give you extremely strong abdominals. As with all planking movements, your legs are major stabilizers here, too.

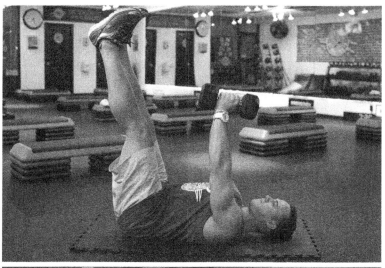

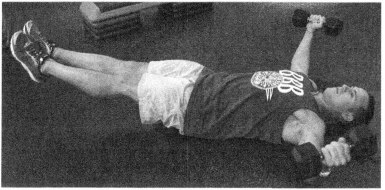

## 5. CHEST FLYES PLUS LEG RAISE *(CHEST AND ABS)*

The chest exercises we choose are for tightening and lifting the chest muscles. Flyes are a great example of this. Like all Better Body movements, we want to get more muscle groups involved. In this case, we are coordinating the arm movement in the dumbbell flyes with the leg movement of the leg raise, to work the abdominals. Not only does this give intense attention to the stomach muscles, but it also slows down the form with the upper-body movement. This forces more control and better results for the chest.

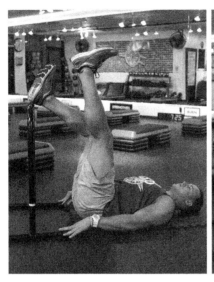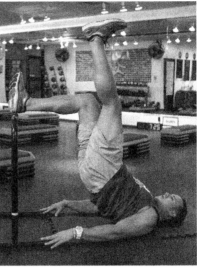

## 6. EQUALIZER GLUTE BRIDGE *(BUTT AND HAMSTRINGS)*

A nice butt isn't built only by working the glute muscles. The hamstrings are also very important because these muscles run all the way down the back of the legs, up and underneath the glutes. Consider strong hamstrings a push-up bra for the booty. These elevated glute bridges give equal attention to both the glutes and the hamstrings. It's one of our secret weapons to building amazing rears for our clients.

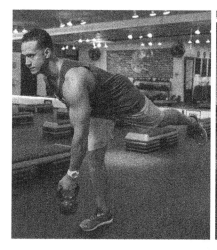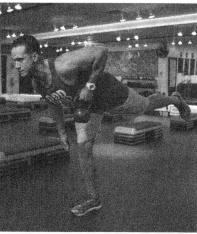

## 7. SINGLE LEG KETTLEBELL ROW
*(BACK, BUTT, HAMSTRINGS, AND LOWER BACK)*

When performing rowing movements from the back, we don't want to work only the upper back. We want to get every rear muscle group into play. For this kettlebell row, we are squeezing the muscles in your upper back slowly with moderate weight to get them tight but not bulky. Many more muscle groups are coming into play here, too. Your obliques are working to prevent you from twisting and tipping over. Your glutes and lower leg muscles are working in overdrive to help you keep your balance. Rounding out the core work, your lower back muscles are also being relied on for stability.

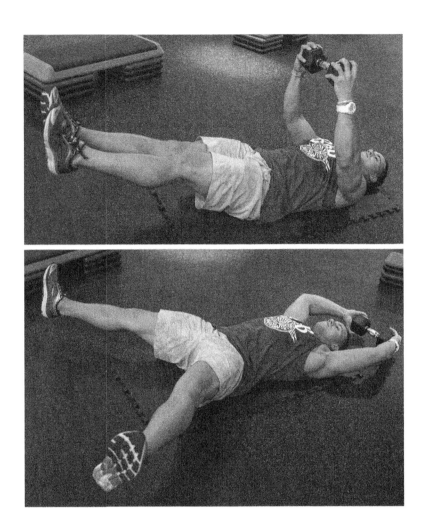

## 8. PULLOVER PLUS SNOW ANGEL *(BACK AND ABS)*

Another great exercise for toning the back is pullovers. This works a specific problem zone for many women: the pocket of fat right in the underarm area. We're combining this with a snow-angel-type movement for the abs. The leg motion shown here will keep the abs working throughout the entire movement, giving you not only a nice back but also a strong and great-looking core.

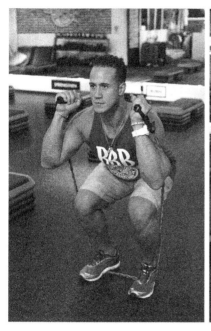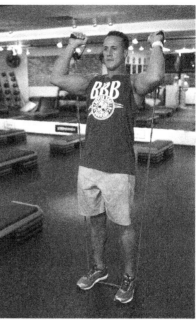

## 9. PUSH PRESS WITH BANDS *(SHOULDERS AND LEGS)*

At Better Body, we like to make upper-body movements full-body movements, and that's no different here with the shoulder press. We're turning this into a push-press, that combines strength from the legs with that of the arms to execute the pushing movement. This exercise is even tougher with bands because the intensity increases astronomically the higher up the arms get in the motion. This achieves great-looking shoulders and legs but also dynamic strength.

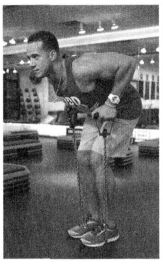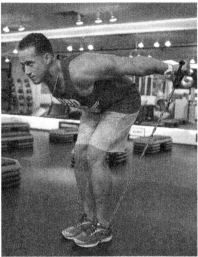

## 10. TRICEPS EXTENSION WITH BANDS *(TRICEPS AND BACK)*

When working the triceps, the small but very important muscles in the back of your arms, we want to bring some major muscle groups into play, too. That's what's achieved with these tricep kickbacks executed with the band. As the triceps are working, the entire upper back maintains a squeeze. This achieves a tight and defined upper back. The bands also are applying resistance to the lower back for stability. So, from the waist up, this exercise is hitting every muscle group in the rear of the body.

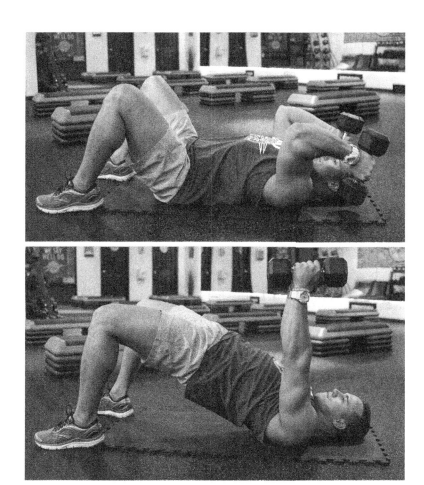

## 11. TRICEPS PLUS GLUTE BRIDGE
*(TRICEPS, BUTT, AND HAMSTRINGS)*

It's a good idea to work your glutes into as many exercises as possible because, let's be honest, they're the first thing anyone checks out on your body. That's what we're doing in this exercise—incorporating a glute bridge into triceps training. Synchronizing the extension of the flexing of the triceps with the slow flexing of the glutes also causes a slower, more controlled, and more intense movement for the arms.

# CHAPTER 5

# FINDING COMMUNITY

I f you're not getting in shape, I would be willing to bet you're lacking community. Either consciously or subconsciously, every single person maintaining excellent shape and living a healthy, vibrant life is taking advantage of community. Don't believe me? Well, let's look closer at what community is all about when it comes to fitness.

It may sound strange, but getting yourself in shape isn't a one-person job. Alone, it's like pushing a rock up a hill with no breaks. It's not fun. But with a community pushing you, it's almost effortless. You have five, ten, twenty, even a hundred people pushing the rock with you, cheering you on, and picking you up when you stumble.

Not only is it easier to get that rock up the hill, it's also a lot more fun along the way, and much more fulfilling once you reach the top.

> **It may sound strange, but getting yourself in shape isn't a one-person job. Alone, it's like pushing a rock up a hill with no breaks. It's not fun. But with a community pushing you, it's almost effortless.**

Those of you taking advantage of community already understand these benefits. For those who have always seen fitness as an individual responsibility that takes a lot of effort, let me offer a quick story about my much younger brother to illustrate my point.

In high school, I was busy, lost in my own world the way most teenagers are. I hadn't paid much attention to my brother's drastic weight gain until I came home from college one summer. To my disbelief, he had ballooned to over 320 pounds! Shocked and concerned, I encouraged him to work out with me all summer. I gave him my weights, bought him a gym membership, and shared nutrition tips and information with him. He loved the initial progress he saw and quickly made friends at the gym. After several months, he lost seventy pounds, put on some muscle, and suddenly, the girls at school were starting to notice him, and the bullying about his weight stopped. With results like that, many of his friends outside his newfound fitness circle also got interested and joined him. Fifteen years later, he has built the body he never thought he could have, maintaining a very lean, ripped 175 pounds.

Results like my brother's are possible for anybody. Having the right friends in high school, or joining a sports team, or having a spouse or partner who encourages fitness training—however it happens, finding a fitness-oriented community—is perhaps the most important component to achieving success in any workout regimen.

If you don't have anyone pushing you to get fit, why not step up and be your own leader? We see it all the time. One spouse or partner will get in phenomenal shape, encouraging the other spouse or partner to enter the gym—admittedly, a little begrudgingly at first. But once that person starts seeing results and begins engaging with this new community, that individual also gets in phenomenal shape. Together, the pair has a new take on life and, inevitably, grows closer from the experience.

Once hooked, some people will make major changes to support their fitness lifestyle. They'll move to a warmer climate where fitness is more prevalent, or they'll change careers so they can dedicate more time to their fitness activities. I don't expect most people to go that far, but your goal should be to get yourself into a community that supports your fitness lifestyle well enough to make it habitual for you. You shouldn't need to make a New Year's resolution. You shouldn't have to put it on your schedule or force yourself to pack your gym bag before work. When you have a good regimen and solid community support, the routine should be automatic and hassle-free.

That's what you want to happen, but of course life is never quite that easy. One obstacle is the people who discourage change. They may be your partying friends from your early twenties, or the shoulder-to-cry-on best friend you had in college. They are dear friends in your adult life, but they may not be the best choices for your fitness life.

**Your goal should be to get yourself into a community that supports your fitness lifestyle well enough to make it habitual for you. You shouldn't need to make a New Year's resolution.**

Your work colleagues may also discourage change, particularly if you work in a sedentary job. Coworkers become, in many ways, your new social circle. These are the people you spend most of your time with, and the habits fostered in that environment eventually become your own. If you have children, the parents of your children's friends are now the people you spend a lot of time with. The point is, you're not making many proactive community choices. That's not good, considering the people you spend your time with are the people you end up being most like. As Jim Rohn once said, "You are the average of the five people you spend the most time with."

It doesn't mean you have to totally cut out of your life people who aren't supporting your fitness. As I always say, how about your being the leader for others? If you don't change your circle in one way or another, you're going to get sucked back into the same lifestyle that got you here in the first place. You have to lead a change among your current community, expand your community, or adopt a new community altogether. That's one of the biggest factors about BBB. I call it our hidden weapon to get in shape, and that's why about 75 percent of what we do is related to the benefits of community.

When someone comes to a BBB gym, chances are they were pulled in by our promises. What they then find is something new, effective, and fun. We have put in years of effort and homework to make this the most effective program in the country. All our knowledge is transferred to the BBB community, but what people value most is how we bring the best out of them. We make our members the centerpiece of the workout by getting to know their hobbies, interests, lifestyles, hopes, fears, and more. The staff we have are exceptional people who take a genuine interest in each of their clients. That's why our company is not running a hundred locations yet.

When new members first come to us, they're partnered with other members. They learn quickly that many of their fellow members are from the same walks of life, which is really a result of the nature of our business. The culture of fitness attracts a certain level of people from around the neighborhood or the kind of people who aspire to do great things with their lives. So, you're surrounded by inspiring people who are at different levels of personal fitness. You may just be starting out and nervous, which makes finding someone else who's going through the same growing pains a great bonding experience. You may meet someone who has been a member for six months and has recently overcome the initial struggles, or perhaps you're drawn to somebody who's been a member for years and is in the kind of stellar physical shape to which you aspire. That's the benefit of the community. You're with goal-oriented people from every level. Some people look to you as a mentor, while you may be looking to others for the same inspiration. You're all sharing a common purpose together.

That's my opinion of what an adult friendship should be. When we were kids, it was about hanging out at the mall or around the neighborhood. Friends were, more or less, just people you passed the time with. But as adults, the words *life is short* begin to resonate more clearly, and we all want to reach our destination more quickly. The gym should bring you into contact with people bound by the same goals and desires to share that same destination.

> **Some people look to you as a mentor, while you may be looking to others for the same inspiration; you're all sharing a common purpose together. That's my opinion of what an adult friendship should be.**

In my opinion, there's no better purpose than getting yourself in shape. I know. Surprising, right? But it's true. Fitness is about living life. It's about not accepting declining health while aging. It's a way to reject the misery, the complaining, the injuries, the lack of confidence, the diseases, and all the other negatives that come along with declining health. It's about refusing to accept stagnation in your relationship and about enjoying being an inspiration to your children. It's about getting out there and not hiding in your house, afraid to go out because you don't feel confident. Fitness is about going out and taking part in the life you want.

I can say firsthand that the BBB community encourages people to get out more. Members find that there's always something to do, whether it's a workout or just a social event. That alone does wonders for people's self-esteem and commitment. The new social circle starts to push you further outside comfort zones, and your routines start to become effortless over time.

The fact that you put some money down and joined something makes it even harder not to show up. Now you have to do it, and if it's done right, you'll want to do it! Having the best techniques, the best equipment, the best coaching, the best people, the most hours, and a highly effective method are all super important in creating the best program; but if you're not there, it doesn't really matter how good the program is. That's where the power of community comes in. We're curating the perfect fitness environment, but the relationships you form with others are what keep you in it.

All of our locations have small staffs, so we have only so much energy. The hundreds of members in that location, however, multiply it. That's the benefit. If you are a BBB member, I'm preaching to the choir. If you're a new member, then you're going to discover this fact soon. But if you're not a member, you need to find a way to get some of these benefits in your own life, and that's what I'm going to teach you here.

## IT STARTS WITH YOU

I'm sure one of your fitness goals is to lose fat, not muscle. Working out is all about feeling stronger, being stronger, and looking stronger, but the results also need to be attractive to you.

The first step is to locate a specialized program that supports your goals in your area. Search the internet and visit the choices that look most promising. They should allow you to have a consultation, and if they don't, or if their consultation is little more than a high-pressure sales pitch, then I would be hesitant. It should be an opportunity to interview the business, and a trial class should be offered. You also want to see if you can join for a month and just observe the level of attention and the overall energy of the place.

There's no perfect program out there, but it should be a place that inspires you. Does it help you get outside yourself? Will it keep you interested? That's what you need to feel out through complementary classes, consultations, or short-term trials. Also, be honest with yourself. Make sure you are giving it your fullest effort but also make sure that the community is meeting you halfway.

Your next step is to be active and social. Get into the outdoors, take up a sport, join a recreational league—whatever it is, stop making fitness a solo activity. Programs such as P90X and Insanity are great. If you're on vacation or home alone, sure, pop in. I always say that more is better. But everything you do should be, at least partly, interactive.

That's where sports activities are helpful. We often find that people come to BBB to burn some fat, get stronger, and become functionally fit. Once they have this new, healthier body, they want to get involved in new things. Obstacle course racing is becoming a popular sport for that reason.

Races are hugely popular because of the community aspect. A race happens every few months and gives you a deadline to train for. When you know your race is coming up in a month, it's going to make you train harder. It's also something to do in a group setting, which brings a competitive edge to it. You want to see how you placed, and you'll come back to try to beat your last record. Knowing that you can do so alongside friends and like-minded people is a bonus.

**We're finding that fitness is the new form of "hanging out." So, instead of grabbing lunch or a drink with a friend, people are taking a yoga class or a kickboxing class together.**

In addition to running and obstacle course racing, we see our members getting involved in all kinds of recreational sports. Many join a soccer, baseball, or basketball league, while others enjoy active sports with less impact, such as tennis or racquetball.

Even as adults, we have a big problem with brainwashing. In Chapter 2, we talked about the broken system created by advertisers that tells us social activity is food based. Instead of playing basketball or tennis, we're more likely to say, "Hey, let's go out for dinner," or, "Hey, let's go to the game and eat hot dogs and chips."

Why not make social activities something different? Instead of going to the game, what if we join a game? These things matter, and we're starting to see a cultural change that shows people's awareness of just how important fitness is. These days, many great companies such as Lululemon have made workout clothing a kind of "going-out" clothing. We're finding that fitness is the new form of "hanging out." So, instead of grabbing lunch or a drink with a friend, people are taking a yoga class or a kickboxing class together. Going out for lunch or a drink afterward is not only more rewarding, but you're also more careful about what you put into the body you just worked so hard on.

So for the next family vacation, let's make it a hike in the outdoors. Instead of grabbing a morning coffee to wake up and chatting with a friend, let's make it a walk or a jog with them instead. For the bonding activities we enjoy at home, let's plan them around healthy cooking. Find a way to do it with other people; don't make it a chore by yourself.

Search for people who will support your fitness lifestyle if you have to. You could strike up a conversation with those fit coworkers you don't talk to very much. Find out where they train. Ask them if they have any hobbies or play any sports, and don't be afraid to ask if you can join. People who take their fitness seriously love to meet others who want to take part in the lifestyle.

If no such person exists in your life, take a class at a local gym and try to meet people there. You can always start by speaking to the class instructor. Where is she working out? What activities does she participate in? You want to make that instructor your friend, which brings us to something else you'll want to know a little about: the nature of socializing at the gym.

## GYM ETIQUETTE

Etiquette isn't too rigid in the fitness world, but it certainly exists. It may not be as complex as attending Easter Mass or as stiff as a black-tie dinner party, but the more you know about basic gym etiquette, the easier it will be to integrate into a particular community.

First off, treat your instructors and trainers with respect. I find too many people treat their instructor or trainer as if that person were a valet or a personal assistant. Instructors and trainers are not your servants. They're there to help you by offering leadership and guidance, so take advantage of it, but do so respectfully. Always thank them after a good class. If it wasn't a good class, thank them anyway and don't go back to the class. Ask them where else they train or what they do personally to stay fit. If you join that gym, at least you'll have someone to say hi to. You might even find someone who can introduce you to some new friends.

Aside from the instructor, make an effort to partner up with people in your class. Be open minded and outgoing. Start saying hi to people and strike up a conversation whenever an opportunity presents itself. **Don't be a wallflower.**

Fitness is the most important part of life, but it's also a metaphor for life. You are not going to get anywhere by being afraid of strangers. Nothing will happen in any area of your life if you don't break out of your shell. In relationships, you're never going to meet the person you really want to meet if you're withdrawn. In your career, you're not getting anywhere unless you're networking. In your community, you're not going to have any influence unless you're active. Your kids are not going to have many other kids to play with unless you're sociable.

And so it goes for fitness, too. Be the leader, say hi, and make a friend. It all goes toward getting your body in shape and creating the kind of life you want.

I can tell you that quality people who have earned their place in life relish the opportunity to mentor, inspire, or simply befriend someone who has a genuine interest in improving. I learned this very early in my fitness career. When I started looking for help, I looked to some of the trainers in my vicinity and was surprised to find that many of them weren't helpful. At first, I thought it was just a dog-eat-dog type of profession, but what I discovered was that when I reached out to the top people in the industry, they were the nicest and friendliest people, such as Gunnar Peterson, who became a friend of mine, and he's still willing to meet me anytime I go to California.

If people aren't willing to help you or don't share these mentoring traits, they could be having a bad day. But if you find they really are just closed-up, selfish people, that tells you a lot about them and their insecurities. Most successful people in the fitness world love to give their very best to those who have a genuine interest. They want to meet people with an enthusiasm for self-improvement; that's what they're in it for. Plus, they didn't get there without others helping them, too.

Even if you feel you are the odd person out, just by going in, introducing yourself, and taking part in the action, you'll find that a good instructor will be more than happy to spend some extra time to help you.

Now, much of what we're talking about in this chapter requires putting money on the line. That can be the moment of truth for people. How much are you willing to invest in your fitness? Fitness must be a core value if you're going to reach your fullest potential. So, start by looking at what else you're spending money on. Clothes, eating out, hair and make up products, tech gadgets? Have those things become core values to you? Probably not, but they may be related to things that are, such as self-worth, friends, and family—or what have you. Your job or career might not be a core value of yours, but the things it helps pay for, such as your family or your leisure, are. When you look at what you spend your money on, you'll find what's most important to you. Spend a little less money on clothes, eat out a little less, and you're going to have money to spend on a gym membership and other fitness-related costs.

Depending on the program, BBB costs anywhere from two to ten times more than a lower-budget gym. But then again, at a lower-cost gym, you're going to be around people who may be less committed, and you'll be stuck in an environment that's not inspired or helpful at all. You get what you pay for, as they say. You may spend ten times as much on us, but we ensure that you get much more than ten times the value.

> **It doesn't take an ounce of hype to say that the time and money invested in your body the way I've described pays you back in both money and well-being.**

Just as with anything today—even walking on the street, breathing, sitting, how you acquired this book—it all costs something. The internet may be free, but the connection costs money. Everything has a price tag somewhere. If you're going to get fit, you'll have to put some money on the line. Find a way to do it, and I guarantee that it will be worth it in the end.

It doesn't take an ounce of hype to say that the time and money invested in your body the way I've described pays you back in both money and well-being. You'll see it in your career when your energy and confidence makes you more productive and generates greater influence. That promotion will be the result of investing in your fitness. Your relationship will be more charged and exciting because you feel better about yourself. Your social life will be more active and fun. Your network of friends and associates will be larger and more diverse. Your health will improve. Simply put, by joining a community and getting fit, the changes extend far beyond the mirror.

Don't just invest in Google or Amazon. Invest in a community. Invest in yourself. That's the investment that's going to pay you back the most.

★ ★ ★ ★ ★ ★ ★ ★ ★ ★ ★ ★ ★ ★ ★ ★ ★ ★ ★ ★ ★ ★ ★ ★ ★ ★ ★ ★ ★ ★ ★ ★ ★ ★ ★

# CHAPTER 5 BBB QUESTIONNAIRE

Answer the questions below to clarify what type of fitness community you want to take part in:

*What are your favorite forms of group activity?*

*Where can you find a fitness community to help support it?*

*Where are there other people in your community that are serious about achieving a better body and life?*

*Where are there group fitness activities that support your desired goals?*

*Is there someone you know that can be a training buddy or accountability partner?*

*How can some of your social activities (quality time with your spouse, playing with your kids, hanging out with your friends) become something fitness related?*

*Where can you find a qualified coach that fits into your budget?*

★ ★ ★ ★ ★ ★ ★ ★ ★ ★ ★ ★ ★ ★ ★ ★ ★ ★ ★ ★ ★ ★ ★ ★ ★ ★ ★ ★ ★ ★ ★ ★ ★ ★

# III

# REPLENISH

# CHAPTER 6

# REPAIRING YOUR RELATIONSHIP WITH FOOD

T here's no discussion about fitness without also discussing food. Food is the fuel that drives our body's progress. If it's used improperly, we get far fewer miles, out of our efforts at best and nothing at worst. Anyone in the fitness field will tell you that food is the most important part of transforming your body. You can't out-train a bad diet, but you can look at what *diet* means a little differently.

This is a book about dispelling the myths and misconceptions surrounding the field of fitness, and I can't think of any area of fitness more riddled with falsehoods than nutrition. For most people, dieting comes with the notion that food is an enemy to your body, and everything but a daily bowl of spinach and gallon of water must be avoided at all costs. This couldn't be more untrue, or unhealthy. If you attack your body issues only from a food angle, you can only approach fitness through calorie deficits and deprivation. How long is anyone going to live like that? And how "fit" will you really be? Skinny is not fit.

**This is a book about dispelling the myths and misconceptions surrounding the field of fitness, and I can't think of any area of fitness more riddled with falsehoods than nutrition.**

Sure, you need to make better food choices, but to do that, you first need to learn more about how food affects your body. After all, no workout is going to counteract your eating a whole box of cookies or a cheeseburger, fries, and a milkshake every day. Not even the best daily workout is designed to burn a 3,000-calorie meal every day.

Fitness counteracts much of the effects, but it can't erase them from your body completely. It can reduce the number of calories resting in your body, but it takes much more work to burn one bad meal than it does to consume it. How much more? Let's look quickly at caloric intake to find out.

## THE CALORIE EFFECT

A BBB workout, or any highly effective workout, will burn a minimum of 500 calories. There are approximately 3,000 calories in a pound, which roughly equates to one fourteen-inch pepperoni pizza or a bacon cheeseburger, fries, a small milkshake, and a large soda. So, just to burn off one or two bad meals (roughly an hour of your time), you'll need to spend about a week working out every day (roughly seven hours of your time).

There is some good news, though. We all know that when you work out, you feel hot afterward. You'll be sweating in your car on the way home, and even after you take a shower, you're still sweating. That's called the afterburn effect. It's the afterburn that you may hear people talking about in the gym. Because your heart rate stays elevated, you burn more calories long after the workout, usually for the next twelve to twenty-four hours. I'm sure you've felt this after a good workout. You're more conscious of your body, more aware of your muscles. You feel hot, energized, and loose. Those calories you burn during the afterburn effect are equal, as a rule of thumb, to whatever you burn in the workout. So, if you burned 500 calories during the workout, you'll actually burn a total of 1,000 calories by the end of the day because of it. That's why, especially in the beginning, a lot of our members will lose a pound every one to three classes, depending on their level of intensity.

Like it, love it, or hate it, food will be a part of your life. Because you can't avoid it, and because we all like to eat something we know we shouldn't every now and again, portion control is one of the best tools you can use to fight the effects of unhealthy eating. Fortunately, working out will make you more conscious of food. Instead of devouring the breadbasket at dinner, you'll say to yourself something such as, "Hey, if I eat one less piece of bread here, I won't negate half the workout I just did."

Maybe you hit your abs hard for a month or two. They're feeling small, you're checking yourself out in the mirror, and you're looking and feeling great. You want more of that feeling, and suddenly that pizza or plate of bacon looks disgusting. It will look bad because you know what it will do to your hard-earned body. You're going to make better food choices. You're going to be a little hungrier, and you should be after a workout, but you'll eventually come to want that feeling. We're supposed to be a little hungry throughout the day. The unnatural thing is to eat so much our stomach expands past our belt size and induces drowsiness.

Getting fit doesn't mean that you can never eat ice cream again. It means you will be more conscious of how much of it you eat and how often. Your subconscious will become your strongest weapon when it comes to moderating your caloric intake. That's the beauty of our brain operating on a reticular activating system.[5] When you're aware of it, you're always aware of it. If you're aware of your body, your calorie burn and consumption, and your performance level, then you're going to be aware of everything that impacts it. You're still going to love where this ends up, however, because you're going to be able to eat whatever you want. I'm not saying it's a good way to go, but by following this book, you won't have to say good-bye to even the worst foods you love.

**Fitness is as much about working out properly as it is about eating correctly.**

## START FRESH

Fitness is as much about working out properly as it is about eating correctly. When your workouts and nutrition are in balance, you get the most visible results but with less energy and time spent achieving them. Trouble is, if you're going to make your life more about fitness and less about food, the odds are already stacked against

---

5    Marilee Sprenger, "How Your Brain Controls Your Attention," Dummies, accessed September 4. 2017, http://www.dummies.com/business/human-resources/employee-relations/how-your-brain-controls-your-attention/.

you. Just turn on the TV and you'll see that life is all about food. Every other commercial is related to food, and a countless number of hours are dedicated to cooking shows or travel programs in which every destination seems to be a restaurant. We're obsessed with eating, and with good reason. We have to eat, but because so much of what we see and hear about food treats it as a source of pleasure, we tend to make bad choices when we do eat.

So, the first thing we need to do is clean out your mental cupboard. You need to forget everything you've heard about the purpose of food before you can repair your relationship with it. You should start by forgiving yourself. Know that the relationship you have with food is not your fault. You're one person in a country of hundreds of millions, many of whom have adopted poor eating patterns. We've all been impacted by the 24/7 messages on television and billboards, in magazines and on social media, many of which indoctrinate us with unrealistic attitudes about food and our bodies. Celebrities who are rail thin are selling you hamburgers, ice cream, and chocolate. Professional athletes are selling you pizza and beer while they rarely, if ever, touch the stuff themselves. It's a manipulation of norms; messages carefully crafted to make you think bad food habits are normal and come without consequences. If we listen to advertisers, we can quite literally have our cake and eat it too.

Culturally, we're built around food as well. Almost every ethnic group prides itself on starchy foods, fatty foods, fried foods, sugary

**The first thing we need to do is clean out your mental cupboard. You need to forget everything you've heard about the purpose of food before you can repair your relationship with it. You should start by forgiving yourself.**

foods, and feasting on large quantities of it. There's nothing wrong with that either. Life was once much more physical than it is today. In fact, virtually all of human life one hundred, or even fewer, years ago was physical and labor intensive. People needed to get together with their family to eat a high-calorie, high-carbohydrate, high-fat meal at the end of the day.

Because the purpose of food was different, its effects were also different. Take carbohydrates for instance. Carbohydrates are the immediate source of energy for our bodies. Your body can store several pounds of them, and if you're physical, that's what it's burning. Your body can also store hundreds of pounds of fat, so if you overeat and the carb stores are full, it's the fat stores that are going to fill up. Because there is an unlimited storage capacity for fat, your body will keep craving food even if you never burn any energy. If we're going to change the effects food has on our body, we have to modernize its purpose in our present lives. Unless you work a labor-intensive job, you simply don't need to consume as much food anymore.

## HURTS SO GOOD

Another strain on our relationship with food today has to do with something a bit darker. It's probably not shocking to hear that we have become an overindulgent society. Technology coupled with an already competitive and hard-working population that's too often short on time has created an on-demand society. We're so accustomed to instant gratification and quick fixes that many of us struggle to accept anything less. Food has become the fallback option for pleasure when we can't find any elsewhere, and when the effects catch up with us, we look to another weakness: overmedicating.

Legal and illegal drug abuse is on the rise. Alcohol abuse is on the rise. Obesity is on the rise, with nearly 65 percent of the population now deemed medically obese. The average American is thirty pounds overweight. Destructive habits and behaviors go hand-in-hand with the mishandling of stress. Dropping an unhealthy habit without replacing it with a healthy one often leads to an even worse problem.

Fixing any self-abuse problem starts with valuing yourself. Looking at yourself in the mirror should feel good. It shouldn't ruin your day or make you want to never leave the house. Ironically, eating is often the go-to activity for when we're feeling depressed, even if we're depressed because of our negative self-image.

But what would happen if the purpose of food was simply not to be hungry? What if instead of a big bowl of ice cream or a thick slice of chocolate cake after a bad day, you used the same time to do a few sets of sit-ups and push-ups? You're getting the same instant release from those feel-good juices in the brain but without the regret and disappointment later. It's a win-win! Plus, a problem certainly won't go away by adding to it.

Leisure is a value of mine. Coming home after a long day and watching some political shows or a silly TV show is something I really enjoy, but I always throw a light workout in there too. It might be a few exercises I missed at the gym or just something to keep my heart rate up, but I've got to stay moving to really enjoy myself. Two or even three hours of watching TV and getting to catch up on pop culture

**Make your time work *for* you rather than against you by integrating your favorite activities with your fitness goals.**

and politics while I work out is a pretty good time to me. If you're home alone, it's a good time to think or reflect on the day. And if you're not, it's something you can do with your spouse or your children too. Make your time work *for* you rather than against you by integrating your favorite activities with your fitness goals. In the process, you'll also be less influenced by any destructive temptations.

We need to get away from the idea of food as a source of fulfillment, because it really isn't. We need to fill it with something else that actually serves us. As I said at the start of this chapter, diets are only about deprivation. Diets are about not eating, eating less, and eating differently. Eating differently is good advice, but let's not deprive ourselves. Let's aim to be full, but let's fill up with other things besides food. Fill up with friends. Fill up with pursuits. Fill up with goals. Fill up with passion projects. Fill up with social activities. Fill up with building a great future. Fill up with love. Whatever it is, don't let food, or anything that's self-destructive, be the only thing you have to fill up with.

Most addicts in recovery relapse because they're bored. And they're bored because they lost both their social circle and the habit they spent most of their time and energy maintaining, because it was their main source of joy. Food abuse is similar in nature. Most of the time we're only eating because we're bored and lacking a feel-good stimulus. We need to find something to fill that gap, and I promise it won't mean cutting out guilt foods completely or banishing our inner foodie.

**Most addicts in recovery relapse because they're bored. And they're bored because they lost both their social circle and the habit they spent most of their time and energy maintaining, because it was their main source of joy. Food abuse is similar in nature.**

★ ★ ★ ★ ★ ★ ★ ★ ★ ★ ★ ★ ★ ★ ★ ★ ★ ★ ★ ★ ★ ★ ★ ★ ★ ★ ★ ★ ★ ★ ★ ★ ★ ★ ★

## CHAPTER 6 BBB QUESTIONNAIRE

Answer the questions below to help clarify your current beliefs about food and how to improve them:

*What are some your negative patterns regarding food? Where are you tripping up?*

*How did these habits develop? How long have you had them?*

*What are some cultural eating patterns you've developed that aren't serving you (American food counts too)?*

*Are you resorting to food to cope in any situations?*

*What can you do instead so that you don't resort to food?*

*What activities are you coupling food consumption with? (For example, before the commute home, beer and alcohol with food on weekends, or high calorie dinners with your spouse.)*

*How can you replace or limit the dependence on food in your social activities or change these activities entirely?*

★ ★ ★ ★ ★ ★ ★ ★ ★ ★ ★ ★ ★ ★ ★ ★ ★ ★ ★ ★ ★ ★ ★ ★ ★ ★ ★ ★ ★ ★ ★ ★ ★ ★

## CHAPTER 7

# FEED YOUR CHANGE: THE POWER OF NUTRITION

**M**ost fitness books leave out nutrition. If they do mention it, it's just a glance and nothing more. A few of the smart programs, though, do make a big deal of nutrition. They realize the importance of it, and we're no different. Performance nutrition, after all, is a big factor in outstanding results.

We know from the last chapter that weight gain and obesity have a lot to do with placing mind over matter. But now that you know why we overeat and how you can make better food choices, *what the heck do we eat*? Let's get into the specifics.

There are a few rules of thumb that I'm going to go over, but first I have to preface this by saying that I'm not a nutritionist, nor a dietician. I do not have a degree in nutrition or dietetics, so I cannot prescribe foods. I can do nothing of the sort, although, as a trainer, I can give advice. Even though I do have a good science background, what's more important for our purposes is that I've spent more than fifteen years transforming the lives and bodies of thousands of members. To me, that experience is like having a doctorate in the school of reality. I know where the nutrition pitfalls are that people most frequently encounter, and my firsthand knowledge of those problems has taught me how to address them.

Nutrition goes beyond just losing weight. It even goes beyond being healthy and preventing diseases. Nutrition is about the techniques, supplements, and ways of eating that will lead to your optimal performance. Like it or not, as a member of BBB—somebody who's going to make fitness a priority every day of the week for the rest of his or her life—you are now, in many ways, an athlete. So, sports nutrition is going to be very important to you.

**In the pages ahead, I'll show you the ideas behind building a Better Body by discussing:**

★ **Protein**
★ **Carbohydrates**
★ **Fiber**
★ **Fats**
★ **Sodium**
★ **Supplements**

## PROTEIN

We can all agree on the importance of protein in performance and fitness results. At BBB, everything we do is focused on working muscles. Muscle is not just essential to everything related to fitness; it's vital to functioning in life. Period. People are not making muscle by sitting around, which is why strength training is critical to building muscle mass.

Ladies, I'm not telling you to get big and bulky. Increasing muscle mass is what forms the shape of your butt, the tone of your thighs and calves, the look of your shoulders, the tone of your upper chest, and, even though you probably don't want a big back, strength training gives you a tight back that has no bra fat as well as great posture. All of those are muscle issues.

Guys, muscle is pretty obvious. You're a big guy already and you're trying to lose weight, I'm assuming, as this isn't a book about body-building and getting huge. We're tackling how to get cut and defined, having the appearance of muscle.

So, what supports muscle? It's protein. From a sports performance perspective, you need protein in every meal and snack in your day. We're going to get into this more, but we need three meals and two to three snacks every day. Protein should be a component in all of them for the rest of your life. There should never be a time for the rest of your days on Earth where there's a meal that does not include a portion of protein. How much can vary, but up to 40 percent or 50 percent of every meal should be protein.

Now, this is not just me talking. Every major food program in pop culture—the Zone Diet, the South Beach Diet, the Mediterranean Diet, and of course, the Atkins Diet—established protein as a vital component to our diet. Some of them, such as Weight Watchers, do talk about calories. But even these days, especially in the men's program for Weight Watchers, they really emphasize protein. They're getting hip to the idea because they realize the effectiveness of protein and strength training to lose weight.

For your muscles to repair and build, you need protein in the bloodstream, and there is no storage area of protein in the body other than in the muscle. In fact, if you do break down muscle and your body has no free amino acids in the bloodstream, your muscles will just continue to break down. You may actually look worse from working out. You'll get a little flabby and feel very weak if you're not supplementing with protein in every meal and snack in your diet.

Protein is the building block of muscle, and because of that, it has gotten a bad rap. When you think of protein shakes or supplementation, you probably think of a body-builder breaking twelve eggs on his weight bench and drinking them down raw, or eating two steaks for every meal. Or maybe you imagine a body builder chugging one of those big protein shakes with God-knows-what in it. We also hear about research studies that link kidney failure and bladder problems to a scientist overdosing lab rats with protein. But I really can't imagine anything that you overdose on that won't have a harmful effect. Everything is about using the right amount.

With protein, you're going to immediately feel stronger, but there are a few things to keep in mind. Protein does not have an immediate energy benefit, unlike carbohydrates, which your body can use as an energy source during exercise. But even if you're not physically active or if you're under a lot of stress, protein will help support your energy level by preserving your muscle. If your muscles are repaired, they're stronger and, obviously, you'll feel stronger, too. If you're feeling stronger, you'll be more active, and if you're more active, you'll have more energy because you're using your muscles more. Protein fuels your fitness lifestyle to come full circle, so if you're feeling weak or stressed, or you're not seeing or feeling an improvement after working out for a few weeks, look at the amount of protein you're consuming.

## CARBOHYDRATES

Beyond sports performance, most nutrition books and nutritionists will deal with protein as a weight loss tool. It truly is a remarkable weight loss tool because most of us gain our unwanted weight through starches. Carbohydrates are the predominant form of calories in almost every type of food today, and they don't provide the nutrition you need. Considering easily consumable, fast, cheap, and tasty foods are so popular with most Americans, it's no surprise that obesity and poor health are growing concerns across the country. The heavy dose of carbs, starches, fats, sugars, and salt found in these foods is a perfect recipe for weight gain and destroying health.

Pure sugar, pure starch, and pure carbs do not exist in nature. Most fruits, for instance, are starchy, and all fruits have carbs. Fruit juices, however, are almost entirely sugars, fats, and carbs because they've broken down the fiber. In many cases, manufacturers mix in more sugar and put it in a form that you can chug and have hundreds upon hundreds of grams of carbs at a time. Even though fruit juice is better than drinking regular soda, it's not much better.

Whole fruit is also frequently used as a dieting tool, making it a common mistake for many of our new members who are trying to eat healthier food and lose weight. They tell me, "I'm eating a lot more fruit. Why am I not losing weight? Why am I gaining weight? I'm having two bananas at breakfast and two oranges and cherries at lunch." They have a diet almost entirely composed of starch without protein, so their sugar is spiking, and the excess carbohydrates are causing the weight gain.

Moreover, these fruits, even though they're natural sources, are generally picked from plants that have been genetically modified over years to have a more popular taste, since tastes evolve as foods and the methods used to prepare them change. If you look at the original versions of these fruits, they're actually much smaller and much more bitter, meaning they don't taste as good to our modern-day palettes.

When our forbearers hunted and gathered their food, ingredients such as sugars, fats, and starches were harder to get in an average diet, and even if they could get them, they took much longer to prepare. That doesn't mean they were healthier, though. Today, people like to point to the so-called glory days of our ancestors living in caves and enjoying great health. That's garbage. I'd take today's society with the risk of overeating over the risk of starvation or being eaten by a saber-tooth tiger or stepped on by a wooly mammoth any day.

> **The human body was not meant to metabolize modern processed foods and the quantities in which we consume them.**

That being said, the human body was not meant to metabolize modern processed foods and the quantities in which we consume them. We live longer, and certain health problems, inevitably, have more time to creep up on us with age, but many of them are induced by our food choices and activity level. When you consume starches in the way we do in modern society—processed, all sugar, pure starch—they shoot your insulin level up in an unnatural way your body was not meant to handle. They put a lot of pressure on your pancreas, the organ that releases insulin, and eventually turn your system haywire. When your body produces too much insulin, the natural amount of sugar that should be in your bloodstream to support your body and your brain isn't there. This overproduction of insulin, which sometimes can be as much as ten times what your body should be producing, will shuttle all the food you ate into your cells. Your cells can't hold all of that excess food—except one type of cell: a fat cell. If your body needs more places to put excess food, it's going to make more fat cells. Your body can produce an almost unlimited amount of fat cells. That's why we see people go up to three, four, five hundred pounds, and beyond. The unfortunate thing is that once a fat cell is made, it can't be destroyed. Fat cells can only be shrunk. So, you've got to be very careful not to make any more fat cells than you already have. Those fat cells that already exist will have to be starved.

So, let's talk about how to play the shrinking game. The goal for your diet is to feed a normal, healthy, and energized life without feeding your fat cells. We want to feed your muscles, your energy level, and even some of the places where your body can hide food without it turning to fat.

To be clear, as with addiction, an almost identical process occurs with bad eating habits: even the smallest morsel of what you eat, a little piece of chocolate perhaps, can have an overwhelming insulin response. So, if you have one piece of chocolate, you end up craving ten more pieces, and you're not satisfied until you have more. As soon as the chocolate is gone, though, because of that violent insulin response, your body is now completely empty of sugar. It was all sucked away into fat cells, so you're feeling drained, sluggish, and hungry a short time later. This is what losing the food game looks and feels like.

What happens on the losing end, when you've got to have more chips, more chocolate, more soda? It's a runaway process that never ends. It's how we get to weigh three, four, five hundred pounds, or even that ten or twenty pounds of unwanted, annoying weight that we can't lose. It's the same type of process.

This runaway hunger effect you may be feeling will subside, however, if you start to eat protein. Protein creates a limited insulin response. Keep in mind, however, that too much protein will create an elevated insulin response because your body has a very easy and simple pathway to turn protein amino acids into sugar. This is why people who go on overly restrictive diets or on starvation diets don't get into shape. It's why they lose both energy and muscle: the body will all too easily break down muscle and turn it into sugar.

The bottom line is, if you're trying to trick, outfight, or deceive your body, which is almost a perfect machine, you're going to lose. If you're trying to starve your body, your body will win. You're not going to want to walk around all day hungry any more than you want to walk around stuffed with soda, pizza, and chocolate. But if we have a balanced diet with a proper amount of fats, proteins, and starches, then we're feeding our energy level, our muscles, and our tummy.

On the subject of starches, there are good starches and bad starches. I've included supporting lists for you at the end of this chapter, but we have to keep in mind the **glycemic index** and the **glycemic load**.

The glycemic index refers to the fact that some sugars are more "sugary" than other sugars, meaning that some of them are very quickly and easily absorbed in your body and will lead to an excessive insulin response.

The glycemic load refers to the total amount of sugar. The perfect examples I like to point to are carrots and cherries. Both of their glycemic indexes are very high, meaning the sugar in them is a sugary sugar. Their glycemic load, however, is low, so there is not much sugar in them overall. The glycemic index is our main concern, though, as it's how we rate a good sugar and a bad sugar. The actual sugar content of cherries, for instance—that's, the amount of sugar you read off the packaging—is not the same amount that hits your body. The actual calorie content is not what hits your body, either.

Potatoes, bread, flour—all of these have a score of nearly 100 in starch.[6] It's not like your test in math class; one hundred is the worst score. It means these foods are pure starch, which results in a pure insulin response.

## FIBER

Fiber, found mostly in veggies and fruits, is going to do a few things for you. It's going to slow the digestion of food and it's going to reduce the insulin response. Of vegetables, organically raised vegetables are full of enormous amounts of essential nutrients. They can have as much as five times the nutrients of nonorganically raised vegetables, so they're going to make you full. Having a large salad with some starch and some protein is a full meal. You're going to be stuffed, and you won't be hungry again for four or five hours. Make use of this information.

Vegetables, especially these days, with healthy salads, with good recipes, through modern agriculture, taste great. Squash, tomatoes, eggplants, zucchinis, cucumbers, beans—they're delicious, and there's a seemingly endless list of ways to prepare and use them. In the beginning, you may not think they're delicious, especially if you're a salt, fat, and sugar eater. Look at it this way: the salad chefs at Wolfgang Puck's have nothing, in terms of skill and resources, on the scientists in the kitchen at McDonald's. The folks in the fast food

6   http://www.glycemicindex.com

labs know better than anyone else how to make you fat and keep you eating.

That being said, once you get off your addiction, a good salad can taste great. Your taste buds will change, and once you repair the sensitivity of your insulin response, the fatty, salty, starchy foods are not going to taste as good anyway.

## FATS

Of all these nutrition hurdles, fat is what I consider the worst. If you do eat out, even if you eat healthy food when you eat out, fat is in the mix. Sorry to break the news to you; it's being masked, and so is the salt. You can eat the healthiest meal at the fanciest restaurant and I promise you that it has more salt and fat than you would like. It's still better than eating the bad food on the menu, so go ahead and eat a healthy meal when you eat out.

Some of the most popular foods—French fries, hamburger buns, pizza crust, for instance—may not have the highest fat content on paper, but they're pure starch and rank among the highest in carbs, which triggers an explosion in insulin production. For that reason, they almost always reach the worst score on the glycemic index. For foods such as French fries and pizza crust, we're looking at possibly 300–400 grams of carbs, an unbelievable amount of carbs. Your body can't stomach that amount, your insulin response is thrown out of whack, and it all ends up being stored as fat.

Ice cream is sugar and fat. Hamburgers are more fat than protein. There's more fat in those fries than in the carbs, so your body is trying to use this increased insulin response to get all of these calories out of your blood and take the high calorie fat with it. The healthy fats are nuts, avocado, olive oil (in moderation), and more. We have a list for you at the end of this chapter.

Fat is very calorie dense, so it's great to keep you full. A little bit of olive oil or an avocado in your salad are excellent sources of sustenance, but unhealthy fats such as cheese are devastating to your diet. It's a shame because it's very easy to overeat cheese. Most restaurants serve cheese as if it's a food on its own, whether it's on bread, chips, or by itself. Unfortunately, cheese is a very saturated form of fat. Okay, it's basically pure fat. What's worse is that it's usually eaten in combination with starches and salt, such as bread or chips, which is the magic recipe to gain weight.

Cheese should really only be used as a seasoning. That's one of the main purposes of cheese—to give something flavor. Maybe you'll have it in a salad, because you do want a little fat in your salad. Picture it. You're having a delicious salad with some olive oil, nuts, an avocado, and some cheese shavings. I'm getting hungry just thinking about it. With a reasonable portion of protein, such as chicken, we have a great nutritious meal. Hopefully I got my workout in for the day and I'm going to be losing weight, which of course is the bottom line in this case.

As we discussed, food is a part of life, so we might as well enjoy it! But on your weekday grind, eat like a Spartan, eat sparingly. Have your go-to meals for breakfast, lunch, and snacks, and have healthy dinners. If you do indulge every now and then, it won't kill you. Even having that occasional pizza dinner won't kill you, which we're going to talk about in the next chapter.

## SODIUM

Now, let's talk about a missing piece here: salt. Salt puts a lot of flavor into food, which, obviously, makes you want to eat more. It elevates the hunger response. So, as if your insulin sensitivity being out of whack wasn't enough, salt makes you even hungrier and thirstier. We've all probably heard the advice about not drinking ocean water if you ever find yourself in the unfortunate position of being lost at sea. The worst thing you could do in that situation is drink the water, because the salt in the water will dehydrate you even more.

If you're eating at Chipotle or McDonald's or wherever, you can see the chunks of salt on the chips and fries, which masquerades the true taste of the food. Your mouth is burning because of the salt, so you eat more and drink more of that sugary soda.

Again, in some ways, it's not your fault. We're surrounded with bad influences and offered very few good options when it comes to proper nutrition and fitness. The ad budgets for fast food companies are in the billions, and you're subconsciously bombarded by such ads. After you have read this book, though, continuing to eat bad food will be your fault. You are armed with the knowledge you need and you are now responsible.

Reducing your salt, sugar, carbs, and fat intake is as simple as introducing more raw vegetables and fruits and lean proteins into your diet.

## SUPPLEMENTS

The final thing I'd like to leave you with is supplementation. Food is anywhere from 50 to 80 percent of the weight-loss game, making what you eat an unquestionably important piece of the fitness puzzle. Your dietary needs can be broken down into two categories: **macronutrients**, such as fats, proteins, and carbohydrates, and **micronutrients**, such as iron, zinc, manganese, and copper. We get most of our macronutrients from the everyday foods we eat, but to ensure we get enough micronutrients in our diet, we need to look elsewhere. That's where we find vitamins and supplements, which are both important to our dietary health and extremely convenient.

The reality is, you need a broad-spectrum **multivitamin** in your diet. Do a little bit of homework and you'll find negative things said about multivitamins. Some people will even say that having a multi is unnecessary if you have a balanced diet, but I couldn't disagree more. Despite our best efforts, most of us do not have a perfectly balanced diet, thus our need for a broad-spectrum multivitamin to supplant that imperfection. A good multivitamin is usually just one pill a day and covers the basics of healthy nutritional input, as well as helping to stabilize energy levels and appetite.

For muscle preservation, there are a few go-to supplements in addition to a multivitamin. Glutamine is the primary amino acid in your muscles. Glutamine is a branch-chain amino acid, meaning it's essentially protein that is already broken down. Glutamine is four times as necessary as any other amino acid. It's an essential building block, so even if you have protein, you'll only build or repair muscle as fast or as much as you have glutamine in your bloodstream.

Usually, protein is anything that was once alive. Amino acids are just the protein completely broken down. **Glutamine** gives you two ways to get aminos. One is from the amino acid profile found in the muscles of the animal (the protein source), and the other is from naturally occurring free aminos. Each aids in muscle repair, so throwing a teaspoon of glutamine into a protein shake will only enhance the amount of protein that actually turns into muscle. Having enough protein in every single meal and snack is going to keep a lot of free amino acids in your bloodstream, but if you want that extra 5 percent strength gain, then glutamine will definitely help you.

For all the benefits they offer, don't buy supplements and think they're going to work magic. If your eating and exercise habits are not in order, there will be no discernible impact from supplements. But if you're eating well and exercising regularly, then making these changes will give you a slight edge.

For those of you out there looking to gain more muscle, **creatine** has been shown to be an excellent strength increaser with minimal side effects. It has a transient effect. This means that as long as you're not taking the creatine, you're going to feel weaker. As long as you are taking it, you're going to feel stronger, thus enabling you to work out longer and harder.

Creatine has been associated with water retention, so if you are taking creatine, it's necessary to have it with some sort of starch. Make a protein smoothie, or maybe something with fruit and a scoop of glutamine, and then add the creatine. That's the best way to combat water retention and put creatine to the best use.

Now, let's talk about **fat burners**. Something that elevates your heart rate to make you burn calories is essentially worthless—and potentially harmful.

A supplement such as ephedra (which is now illegal) worked by keeping your heart beating faster so your body would think it was jogging, a confusion that could help burn an extra 250 calories in a day. Trouble is, you put an unnatural strain on your cardiovascular system and heighten your chances for a heart attack or other serious medical conditions.

A fat burner really has no place in a normal person's weight-loss regimen. That also goes for many "pump" drinks and nitric oxide drinks, which are often mixed with sugar and are pumped straight into your bloodstream. They're meant to cause vasodilation and make you want to work out, but that's garbage. Just warm up a little bit and you're going to want to work out.

This process of keeping yourself in the best shape possible is a lifelong commitment. Supplements can help, but they can't do it all for you. They're not entirely necessary, but if you're doing everything else right, have at it. They will certainly help you get the best results from your fitness regimen.

The goal is to eat the right things without feeling deprived of anything. It's about working out regularly while still maintaining a normal life. Ideally, you'll be eating delicious, healthy foods at the right times, in the right proportions, and feeling energized and happy all the time because of it. Your diet fuels your body, which in turn fuels your fitness. And your fitness, as we all know, fuels a better life. For that reason, the importance of eating correctly can't be overstated. So, whether you're starting over, starting from scratch, or rekindling the relationship between your fitness and your food, just know that reimagining the purpose of food as a tool to transform your body will cut down the amount of time you spend sweating in the gym and deliver bigger, better results faster and more easily. Sound worth it? I think so.

## NUTRIENT TIMING

We talked about the importance of protein in your snacks and meals, but your timing in consuming them is just as important. On a cellular level, muscles are more receptive to nutrients after a workout because they're craving nutrients to repair themselves. Thinking of nutrition in terms of your physical performance requires you to keep in mind key periods when your body will digest nutrients and make the most use of them. Right after your workout is the most vital window for consuming essential nutrients. This absorption phase is key phase for your body's transformation. Absorption refers to the time when your body is most actively delegating the foods you eat toward muscle repair and replenishing energy stores.

## EAT WHATEVER THE HECK YOU WANT

Now that you know what all of the macronutrients are, let's put them together into a plan that will help you burn fat, serve your workouts and energy level, and also be very easy to follow. I call it the "eat whatever the heck you want" plan.

The reason that most diets fail is because they're too restrictive. Some plans call for no carbohydrates, ignoring that most common foods we enjoy contain carbs (and also ignoring that carbs are essential for a strong metabolism and energy level).

> Let's put them together into a plan that will help you burn fat, serve your workouts and energy level, and also be very easy to follow. I call it the "eat whatever the heck you want" plan.

Other plans have you eating far fewer calories than you require. This is also a failing formula. Undereating by too much will cause you to dump lean muscle, decrease your energy, ruin your mood, and inevitably cause a rebound where you eat more and gain more weight than ever.

A better strategy is nutrient timing. That means having your macronutrients at times they best serve you. At these times, they're more likely to be used for energy and body repair, rather than stored as fat.

Also part of the "eat whatever the heck you want" plan is finding times where you can eat some of your "cheat" foods so that they don't ruin your results. What I think you'll find is that once you adopt an eating strategy and are consciously working to execute it, you'll eventually wean yourself off of cheat foods and never have to rely on them again.

Here is your food chart. The portions and timing here are in line with every major diet program out there, not to mention the leading research on weight loss and weight management. A key part of this plan is smaller, more frequent meals. An explanation of each element of the plan will be included later on in this chapter. You'll also get a full list of the good, better, and best foods to incorporate into your plan at the end of this chapter.

Before we break down each of the meals individually, let's talk about the plan as a whole. The mistakes that can be made with this plan have to do with the number of meals that are on this chart.

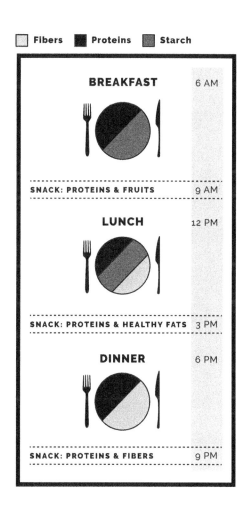

When adopting this new plan, some people keep their meal sizes the same and then just add more snacks. This will of course cause you to gain more weight because you have increased your overall food consumption. That's why if you're currently eating only two or three meals, a good rule of thumb is to cut the portion sizes of each of these meals in half and then incorporate your snacks from there. A snack should be about half the size of one of your meals. In the beginning, cutting your meal sizes this much may require some willpower, and you'll find yourself a little hungry. Eventually, you'll find your calorie needs at each meal decrease, and you'll never find yourself overeating again.

## BREAKFAST

 **BREAKFAST**  6 AM  With breakfast, you'll find half of your plate consists of protein and the other half is carbs. You'll be having your carbs early in the day to give you plenty of fuel to burn for energy. Protein is what supports your muscle strength and repair and can also be burned for energy. Calorie-wise, breakfast should be your biggest meal of the day. For those of you that currently skip breakfast, this will take some getting used to. You can start with eating just a small meal that's half protein and carbs to start, and build up from there.

## SNACK #1

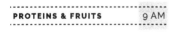 **PROTEINS & FRUITS**  9 AM  Your first snack of the day follows the same game plan as breakfast. You can enjoy carbs all through the early part of the day and balance it with protein to keep your muscles strong. Remember, your snacks

are about half the size of a small meal, but since you're eating through the day, you'll never feel hungry. You'll find a small piece of fruit recommended above as your carbohydrate. For protein, check the chart at the end of this chapter for something of your choosing (a protein shake works with your snacks too).

## LUNCH

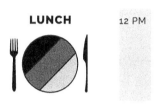

LUNCH    12 PM

The macronutrients of lunch look very similar to breakfast. Your plate will consist of an equal portion of protein and carbs. The big difference is this meal also has an equal portion of fiber, which means vegetables. Although you have a full plate of delicious food, your calories in this meal will be less than they were at breakfast because fibrous foods have a negligible amount of calories.

## SNACK #2

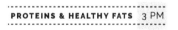

PROTEINS & HEALTHY FATS   3 PM

After lunch, we are starting to curtail carbohydrate consumption for the day. The reason is that carbohydrates are a good source of immediate energy for the busier, more active parts of your day. Having them closer to bedtime, when you are totally inactive, will increase the chance that your carbohydrate stores will be full, and everything above that will be stored as fat. If you still need to have carbs later in the day, there are some exceptions; we'll discuss this at the end of this chapter. However, you won't be starving yourself late in the day. You can still enjoy healthy fats, which you'll find examples of in your food chart at the end of this chapter. And you can also fill your plate with fiber, which you'll find at dinner time.

## DINNER

**DINNER**   6 PM

We're now at the tail end of the day. The good news is you've been eating small meals and snacks every few hours, all day. That means your hunger should be decreasing by the end of the day. If you're the type of person that wasn't eating much at all during the day (which is what most busy people do these days), this may have been the opposite. What most people find themselves doing is overeating at the end of the day, with much of that food being stored as fat while they sleep. To make matters worse, since you weren't eating through the day, your body was burning your muscles for fuel all day. This new plan will keep you burning fat and carbs for energy all day and during your workouts.

## LATE SNACK

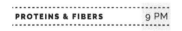

**PROTEINS & FIBERS**   9 PM

Depending on when you eat dinner or when you go to bed, you may need a late-night snack. This will help preserve muscle while you sleep and also curb your appetite come time for breakfast. Chances are, you're going to feel very satisfied and stress-free after a day of energizing and healthy eating. If you still find yourself resorting to sweets late at night, which is a habit for many people, we'll get into some solutions at the end of this chapter.

Fat is healthy but very high in calories, so the amount you consume should be carefully watched and eaten in negligible quantities. The saturated fats in a lot of foods can actually cause fatal health issues.

## THE ROAD TO PERFECT EATING

What you'll find in the eating plan above was a discussion of the macronutrients (protein, carbs, fibers, and fats) to eat. We didn't get into exactly what foods to eat. For you, this can be a personal decision. You can eat the foods you already like to eat as long as they are consumed at the appropriate times and in the portions we're talking.

For protein shakes, you can pick any brand you want, or avoid them altogether if you prefer to replace them with real food instead. With whatever shake you choose, or when mixing it yourself, find one that doesn't have any carbohydrates added. If you are mixing the shake with a carbohydrate base or adding fruit, keep in mind that this will affect the macronutrients on your chart.

The road to better eating starts with the foods you're already eating now. You don't have to do anything drastic by changing everything about your diet. However, once you're eating smaller meals more frequently and in the right portion sizes, you can start to improve the quality of these foods.

That's the plan. Start eating in the right portions at the right times, and you'll start enjoying the energizing and weight-loss benefits. After that, just like each of your workouts will get better, you'll find the specific foods you're eating getting better, too.

## SOLUTIONS SHEET

In consulting with countless clients over the years, I've noticed a pattern of where they're tripping up with their eating. It's surprising how many people have the same bad eating habits. Luckily, there are easy-to-follow solutions for all of them. Here are solutions to some of the common ones below:

**PROBLEM:** The morning bagel.

**SOLUTION:** A bagel is one of the largest and most common carbohydrate meals (others are waffles, croissants or pancakes). The simple solution is not to change any of the foods in the beginning. The trick is simply to cut the portion of carbs here by a half or more and add protein to the meal. By making half the meal protein, you haven't cut your calories at all. You've only made the meal less likely to make you fat. Protein also fills your stomach and makes you less hungry than carbohydrates, so you should be able to eat fewer total calories for breakfast without feeling hungry at all. And if you're a big breakfast eater and aren't happy that you have to cut the size of this meal, don't worry; you have a snack coming up in only three hours.

**PROBLEM:** Sugar in your coffee.

**SOLUTION:** Pure sugar sources are obviously something you want to eliminate from your diet. But cutting sugar in your coffee doesn't have to be done cold-turkey. At first, cut your sugar quantity in half and replace it with the artificial sweetener of your choice. Continue to decrease the amount of sugar. You'll soon find that you're not relying on sugar at all. After that, you can slowly cut your amount of artificial sweetener and may be able to get away with very little or none of that, too.

**PROBLEM: Sweets or ice cream at night.**

**SOLUTION:** This has got to be the biggest cheat I hear about. The reason for it is, I think, most people aren't eating enough throughout the day. If you've had a stressful day where you haven't eaten through most of it, you lose control by the end of the day. You're just looking for as many calories and any type of comfort food you can get your hands on. This can first be solved by sticking to your eating plan through the day. Because you have fueled your body through the day, you'll find your cravings decrease at night. If you're still craving sweets and fat and at night, the first alternative to wean yourself off the habit can be purchasing low-carb versions of popular sugar products. They don't taste quite as good but can satisfy your cravings. There's also another big benefit: You don't get the same insulin spike that sugary products give you. That means you won't crave more of it, and you will eventually become free of the metabolic addiction these sugary foods were giving you. The Atkins food company makes dozens of varieties of low-carb candy bars that you can chose from to satisfy your sweet tooth. There are also numerous other companies that make cookies and even ice cream in a low-carb form. Although these low-carb products have ingredients that are of questionable health benefit, our goal is not to be eating them forever. It's to simply break the late-night craving addiction, which should happen after only a few weeks. Another option is peanut butter or almond butter and celery sticks. If you've never tried them, they're delicious. The fat from the nut butter will please your taste buds, and the fiber from the celery will fill up your stomach.

**PROBLEM: Soda, juices, and alcohol.**

**SOLUTION:** The sugar in drinks like soda, juice, and alcoholic beverages can be the biggest fat-loss killer. Chances are, you have to quit cold-turkey, and with alcohol, drastically cut the amount you're drinking, or switch to lower calorie drinks. When it comes to sugary drinks, if cold-turkey doesn't work, you can try to substitute at first. For sodas, many of them now come with natural artificial sweeteners. No matter what, diet soda is of highly questionable nutritional value, so our goal in drinking them is to simply break the addiction. For juices, you can also take the same approach and drink flavored diet drinks like Crystal Light. But the goal is to stop drinking any artificial drinks all together. When it comes to alcohol, you're not in college anymore, so it's time to lay off of the beer and the weekend drinking binges. If wine at dinner is your vice, try to keep it to only one glass. You'll want to make sure your dinner has no carbs as we described with our food chart above. And you're going to have to train hard to burn off those calories!

**PROBLEM: Snacking with your kids.**

**SOLUTION:** The great part about eating healthier yourself is that your family will follow suit. It's much easier to lead your children to a healthier lifestyle when you're setting the example yourself. But children do love their snack foods, and as a parent, you may join in, too. The thing to keep in mind is that all snack foods are loaded with carbs (along with numerous artificial ingredients).

If you are consuming these additional snack carbs, remember to remove them from your meals or snacks. This way, you won't experience a net increase in your carbs for the day. However, don't take your eyes off of the goal: replacing unhealthy snacks with natural, real-food alternatives.

**PROBLEM: Carbs at dinner.**

**SOLUTION:** For some of us, having carbs at dinner-time has been a tradition our entire lives, and it's going to be very difficult to change. It may be a family or cultural habit that's ingrained in you from childhood to adulthood. When it comes to my eating advice, I'm always a realist. I understand that eliminating something you've been doing your entire life may be next to impossible. After encouraging you train more and join new communities throughout this book, I'm not also going to take away what may be a treasured family custom. Instead, let's look at some solutions. The key here will be to replace as much of your plate with protein and fiber as possible. If you are having rice, pasta, or potatoes as part of dinner, make it the absolute minimum quantity. Most of your plate will be filled with the lean protein of your choosing, and vegetables. In this way, your dinner plate will look a lot like your lunch plate. While this meal isn't perfect according to our plan above, it is still a small one. You've been eating all day, so you won't have the desire to binge on carbs at dinner. If you're having an early dinner, according to our eating plan, you'll still have room for one more late night protein snack, so do your best to keep the carbs out of your dinner most nights of the week. But if you're finding this impossible, you don't have to abstain completely. There's also good news if you're a person that trains in the evening. Your glycogen stores are likely to be emptied out after your workout, right around dinner time. So, as long as your dinner is small and sensible, it can still include some carbohydrates without them being stored as fat. Instead, they'll replace the glycogen you burned during your workout.

## YOUR POST-WORKOUT MEAL

The one place where you want to use your judgment in regard to the eating plan is when it comes to your post-workout meal. As you noted on the chart above, we have breakfast as the biggest meal of the day. This is to start your day with a burst of energy and maintain that energy throughout the day. However, these days, many people are training after work or even later at night. At that point, your food intake is starting to drop down, and your immediate energy may drop down, too. If you work out later in the day when not much food is involved, you may want to skew the chart to account for this. While the dinner meal and late snack are the smallest of the day, if you just worked out, you can go slightly larger with those meals. After you train, your body is the most receptive to nutrients and the most likely to use your food for recovery, rather than storing it as fat. So, on the days that you do train late in the day, you can cut some of the food from breakfast and lunch, and add it to dinner. However, I find many of our Better Body members use the eating chart even if they do train at night. While they aren't eating big at night, they are still eating, so their bodies are still getting plenty of calories to recover. It's your personal choice on how to adjust your meal sizes based on when you workout. Just remember to be consistent, and also be sensible. A late-night workout isn't a license to have a burger and fries for dinner!

# THE MAGIC OF INTERMITTENT FASTING

There's an eating trend that's catching on now called intermittent fasting.[7] In a very basic nutshell, it's a weight loss strategy where you go for periods of twenty-four hours or more without eating any food. Many people are swearing by it, and there's a lot of great research pointing to its benefits. Instead of going into a very long discussion of intermittent fasting, let's talk about some ways to use the strategies immediately to keep your eating plan and weight loss or weight management on track.

I use intermittent fasting to counteract some of the inevitable hiccups that can happen in a normal healthy eating schedule. It's how you can prepare for a period of big eating, such as Thanksgiving or Christmas dinner. Or it's how you can recover from a period where you ate too much food, such as a game where you ate too much or a night out drinking where you lost control and hit the diner afterwards.

If you are preparing for a big meal, then you may want to skip a few meals leading up to it. In addition, you may also want to get in a big workout. Once your big meal comes up, your body will re-feed, replacing some of your glycogen stores and using the food for recovery. It's less likely to be stored as fat. And just to be safe, you may want to follow up the big meal by skipping another couple of meals. You may be so full and satiated that you won't even need it. So, overall, the result will be that you haven't consumed any extra calories out of the ordinary. And if you fall back into your normal eating plan, you'll be right back on track to achieve and maintain the best shape of your life.

---

7    http://www.precisionnutrition.com/intermittent-fasting

For the unplanned times when you eat too much, intermittent fasting can work, too. Just like I described, skip the next few meals, and get a good workout in. You want to deplete your energy stores so that no additional food is stored as fat, and the period of fasting along with a good workout will do that.

How long should you fast for? You can use your judgment on that. Skipping a half day of eating should do the trick. You can choose to do more, but don't get so hungry or out of energy that your workouts are affected or that you end up eating another big meal. After a period of fasting, you want to fall right back into your normal eating schedule.

The magic of intermittent fasting is that you may actually end up burning *more* fat and getting more lean than had you not fasted at all. When you have a normal eating schedule, your body is always burning fat and calories through the day. You end up with a high metabolism. So, when your body faces a period without food, it still maintains the calorie burn for a time in spite of it. You'll find you lose the most fat during your periods of intermittent fasting.

However, too many periods without food is called starving yourself, and that has never worked as a long-term solution for someone trying to maintain a happy life full of energy and strength.

A bad meal once in a while is an excuse most people use to completely fall off the wagon. With intermittent fasting, you'll be able to use these cheat meals as a way to burn off even more fat.

## SUMMARY

With a good eating plan, losing a lot of body fat initially is actually quite easy. We see it all the time here at Better Body. And as you just learned with intermittent fasting, even making some mistakes once in a while won't get in the way. It's multiple mistakes over a long period of time, combined with a lack of consistent activity, that will get you in trouble. Remember that your eating plan will take as much effort as your workout plan. It's something that you need to keep reminding yourself of every day, and it will get better over time with practice.

|  | CARBS | PROTEINS | FATS |
|---|---|---|---|
| **A+ FOODS** **BEST** | Spinach<br>Kale<br>Broccoli<br>Brussel sprouts<br>Asparagus<br>Collard greens<br>Red pepper<br>Tomatoes<br>Lentils<br>Alfalfa sprouts<br>Onions<br>Field greens<br>Butternut squash<br>Radishes<br>Bok choy<br>Green beans<br>Spaghetti squash<br>Beets<br>Cabbage<br>Eggplant<br>Green peppers<br>Yellow peppers<br>Romaine lettuce<br>Shirataki noodles<br>Ezekiel bread<br>Gluten free oatmeal<br>Quinoa | Salmon<br>Rainbow trout<br>Herrings<br>Egg whites<br>Whey protein<br>Buffalo<br>Ahi<br>Tuna<br>Cod<br>Tofu<br>Venison<br>Tilapia<br>Orange roughy<br>Mahi mahi<br>Sword fish<br>Perch<br>Sea bass<br>Halibut | Almonds<br>Cashews<br>Avocado<br>Krill oil<br>Flaxseed oil<br>Udo's choice oil blend<br>Fish fat |
| **A FOODS** **GOOD** | Jicama<br>Celery<br>Spring mix salad<br>White potatoes<br>Red potatoes<br>Brown rice<br>Plain oatmeal<br>Yams<br>Sweet potatoes | Ground turkey<br>Non-fat greek yogurt<br>Chicken breast<br>Turkey breast<br>Fish<br>Shellfish<br>Non-fat cottage cheese<br>Top round steak | Olive oil<br>Canola<br>Peanut butter<br>Nuts |
| **B FOODS** **OK** | CARBS<br>100% whole grain<br>cereal<br>100% whole grain<br>pastas<br>100% whole grain<br>bread<br>whole grain pitas<br>whole grain muffins<br>grits<br>cream of rice<br>white rice | Pork tenderloin<br>Flank steak<br>Extra lean top sirloin<br>Low fat sliced turkey<br>Non-fat sour cream<br>Non-fat cheese<br>Non-fat cream cheese<br>Low fat cottage cheese |  |
| **C FOODS** **NOT GOOD** | Pasta<br>Bagels<br>Cheerios<br>Instant oatmeal<br>Kellog raisin bran<br>Total cereal<br>Wheat bread<br>Unsweetened fruit<br>juice<br>Low fat yogurt | Sliced low fat ham<br>Low fat sausage<br>Ground beef<br>Chicken thighs<br>Turkey, dark meat<br>Turkey, ostrich<br>2% cream cheese<br>2% cottage cheese<br>2% sour cream |  |
| **D FOODS** **NOT ACCEPTABLE** | Alcohol<br>Boxed food<br>Pre-prepared foods<br>Fast food<br>Sweetened box cereal<br>Enriched white bread<br>Crackers, muffins and<br>baked goods | Ground beef<br>Fat cut meat<br>Roast beef<br>Ham | Sour cream<br>Cottage cheese |

# GROCERY STORE SHOPPING LIST

## PROTEINS

Buffalo
Venison
Ground turkey
Shrimp
Orange roughy
Perch
Ahi
Boneless skinless chicken
Turkey breast
Lean red meats
 · Flank steak
 · London broil
 · Top sirloin
 · 4% ground beef
Fish
 · tuna
 · halibut
 · sea bass
 · tilapia
 · mahi mahi
 · red snapper
 · shark steak
 · salmon (in moderation)
 · egg whites
 · swordfish

## GOOD FATS

Almonds
Peanuts
Flaxseed and olive oil
Peanut butter
Avocados
Pam and utter spray
Udos oil
Krill oil

## POLY UN-SATURATED FAT

Safflower
Sunflower
Soybean
Corn
Cottonseed

## MONO UN-SATURATED FAT

Olive oil
Canola oil
Peanut oil
Avocados

## DAIRY

Lowfat goat cheese
Sugar free coffee creamer
Almond milk
Soy milk
Greek yogurt
Non-fat sour cream
2% non-fat cottage cheese
Dannon light & fit yogurt
fat free milk (in moderation)

## COMPLEX/STARCHY CARBOHYDRATES

Kashi GoLean
Gluten free
Sweet potatoes
Cream of rice
Quinoa
Rye bread
Ezekiel
Grits
Oatmeal
Red potatoes
Yams
Brown/white rice (in moderation)
Whole wheat pasta
Whole wheat bread
Cream of wheat

## FIBROUS CARBOHYDRATES

Spaghetti squash
Celery
Spring mix salad
Butternut squash
Broccoli
Asparagus
Spinach
Green beans
Brussel sprouts
Cabbage
Cauliflower     Zucchini
Onions          Tomatoes
Mushrooms       Squash
Eggplants       Alfalfa
Bok choy        Cucumber
Lettuce
Artichokes
Jicama

## RECOMMENDED BEVERAGES:

- Water
- Crystal light
- Green tea
- Coffee
- Iced tea (no sugar added)
- Herbal teas
- Almond milk
- Soy milk

## RECOMMENDED BEANS (CARB):

- Black beans
- Kidney beas
- Lentils
- Pinto beans
- Lima beans

## RECOMMENDED CONDIMENTS:

- Ketchup
- Mustard
- Worcestershire sauce
- Light sodium soy sauce
- Balsamic vinegar
- Non fat sour cream
- Fat free mayo
- Relish
- Sugar free mayo
- Sugar free syrup
- Lemon and lime juice
- I can't believe its not butter spray
- Stevia
- Ginger
- Cinnamon
- Nutmeg
- Sage
- Thyme
- Rosemary

## RECOMMENDED SEASONINGS:

- Ms. Dash
- Garlic
- Basil
- Oregano
- Pepper
- Sea salt
- Onion
- Parsley
- Dill
- Cayenne
- Paprika
- Cumin
- Curry
- Dry mustard
- Cilantro

## SERVING PORTION SIZES

### WOMEN

- ½ cup oatmeal
- ½ cup brown rice
- 5 ½ oz. red potato
- 5 oz. sweet potato
- 2 cups of veggies
- 3 oz. protein
- 3-5 egg white
- 1-2 slices of Ezekiel bread
- 3 oz. whole grain pasta

## SERVING PORTION SIZES

### MEN

- 1 cup oatmeal
- 1 cup brown rice
- 8 oz. red potato
- 7.5 oz. sweet potato
- 3 cups veggies
- 5-6 oz. protein
- 7-10 egg whites
- 2 slices of bread
- 5 oz. whole grain pasta

## FRUITS LIST:

### A+ FRUITS
Raspberries
Blackberries
Cranberries
Rhubarb

### B FRUITS
Strawberries
Melons
Papaya
Watermelon
Peaches
Nectarines
Blueberries
Cantaloupe
Honeydew
Apples
Guava
Apricots
Grapefruit
Plums
Figs
Pears

### C- FRUITS
Oranges
Kiwi
Pineapple

### D FRUITS
Tangerines
Cherries
Grapes
Pomegranates
Mangos
Bananas
Dried fruit – dates, raisins,
apricots, prunes

## SNACKS LIST:

94% FF Popcorn
Sugar free pudding
Sugar free jello
Carrot or celery sticks
Rice cakes
Sugar free popsicles
Protein pudding
Hummus
Non-fat yogurt

## LOW-CARB PROTEIN BARS:

Think Thin bites
Permalean bars
Luna Bars
Lara Bars

## LOW-FAT PROTEIN BARS

Promax
Power Bar
Kashi Roll

# REFRESH

**E**verything in this book is an introduction to the techniques and philosophies behind BBB. Of course, at BBB we spend thirty days making changes to your fitness program by gradually increasing the intensity of your workout, tweaking your nutritional intake, addressing your lifestyle challenges, and more, so that we can find your personal sweet spot for getting you where you want to go.

We use a lot of the information in this book to completely rewire the way people look at fitness. When people change the way they look at exercise and food, they inevitably change their results. You will discover that this is an entire metaphor for life. So, as your fitness journey progresses, so too will your life.

> **We use a lot of the information in this book to completely rewire the way people look at fitness. When people change the way they look at exercise and food, they inevitably change their results.**

Through your fitness, you really are fixing your life. Treat it with that level of importance and you will find so much more than a slimmer, toner body in the mirror.

I believe one of humankind's great discoveries was that we have control over our lives. I think it's a modern thing, especially in America, to appreciate self-reliance and zeal, to praise one's commitment to progress, exploration, and personal improvement, no matter the odds. Such values are incredible tools. They make possible one's journey of self-discovery and enlightenment in the pursuit of a better way of life. But I'll be honest. I am not a believer in the self-help movement. I have found that most of it is a lot of talk with very little action. I do, however, like the primary idea behind it: We can change.

So, let me say this to you now: Your body *can* change. You are not chained to it. You are not forever doomed to live the way you are living now. Many areas of your life are fixable. We have the ability to change our thoughts, our careers, our relationships, and perhaps more easily, we have the ability to change our eating habits and our bodies.

> **Your body *can* change. You are not chained to it. You are not forever doomed to live the way you are living now.**

How do you go about doing that? It's not through mantras and positive self-talk, although that does help. It's not necessarily goal-setting either, although that definitely helps, as well. And it's not just your social circle, either.

Unlike most self-help subjects—your mind, your job, your marriage, your parenting, and so on—the body is something concrete, something visual. You can see the changes happening. Fitness-related changes are measurable, either by the amount of time you can run, the weights you can lift, the times you go to the gym, the size of your clothes, or just the numbers on your scale. It's a very physical meta-morphosis, so we have a way to transform your life that's very specific, one that acts as a vehicle for major life changes and has the metrics to prove it. We have a real physical indication, whether it's in the mirror, our interpersonal interactions, the removal of physical limitations, or in our wardrobe. We have given ourselves a goal, and we can see and feel our successes every day just by pursuing it.

**You can see the changes happening. Fitness-related changes are measurable, either by the amount of time you can run, the weights you can lift, the times you go to the gym, the size of your clothes, or just the numbers on your scale.**

Someone once told me that all we really need in life is a game worth playing. Many of us are just kind of wandering around, not sure what to do because we don't feel that we have a game worth playing, something to just dive into and allow ourselves to be consumed by. Some of us pour ourselves into work. Some of us rely on a relationship. But workaholics are not healthy or happy, and I'm sure we've all had the experience of being in a relationship with someone who was too needy. We hear of people all the time who were burdened with overbearing parents, too.

But when it comes to your body, diving in is something you can't overdo short of an eating disorder or supplement abuse. Fitness is going to be something positive in your life, something that serves you and those who care about you.

So, following what we discussed in this book—by planning and prioritizing your workouts, saying no to certain foods and eating habits, and putting yourself first—you will immediately be on your way to healthier self-esteem and greater self-confidence.

Too many people look at life as a grueling chore. Consequently, they look at fitness the same way. As does life, fitness needs to be fun. You need to look forward to it, and the only way to do that is to take control and prove to yourself that getting fit is full of positive results if you put the work in. Pursue the things in life that serve you, that make you better, that make you a person of more influence by aligning with your values. Be a person you would like to be around, someone who feels good about life and enjoys living. That's what we're going to discover through fitness. And now that you have a plan, you can tackle your body in a new and effective way.

You have the opportunity to add a new pursuit to your life, one that will make achieving everything else you want that much easier. Giving your body the attention it deserves will lay the foundation for the life you deserve. So, start your Better Body revolution today. Really. Start right now. You can reach higher, and you can achieve it!

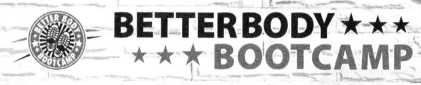

# BETTER BODY ★ ★ ★
# ★ ★ ★ BOOTCAMP

## OUR SERVICES

At **Better Body Bootcamp,** we help our members get leaner and look better, and, as a result, live healthier, more fulfilling, and more confident lives through group training services for women and men of all ages. Our difference is in a revolutionary approach that combines strength training exercises specifi-cally chosen to tone and sculpt you, rather than bulk you. This is always combined with high intensity cardio, creating a fat-burning interval pace, from the first minute of our classes to the last. The best part of all is that our training happens in a fun and friendly group environment with people on the same mission as you. What results is a fitness community, lasting friendships, and a positive impact on our surrounding neighborhoods.

**To begin the journey of discovering your own unlimited potential, find a Better Body location near you at**

# www.betterbodybootcamp.com

CPSIA information can be obtained
at www.ICGtesting.com
Printed in the USA
BVOW09s0919271017

498822BV00018B/396/P

# WHAT MARK'S ADVOCATES

The Time Mastery System has been life ch̶ ̶.ally. What might look like to some as a "to̶ ̶. effective plan for taking back control of your day. ̶ back control, you are no longer bogged down by the tas̶ take your valuable time away. You begin reaping the benefits on the first day, but its true results manifest themselves weeks down the road. I now have the time to focus on the "long-term" objectives, or the "improving myself" items that always seemed to get pushed off until tomorrow. Try it. Stay with it. Change your life!

**JIM REARDON**
*Production Manager*
*RI Kitchen & Bath Inc.*

I have been using Mark's Mastering Time for several months now. Not only does it help me whittle time from my day by staying on track, but it also helps me leave my day feeling more accomplished. I couldn't live without it now and would encourage anyone to give it try.

**JENN HARBICK**
*The Neil Kelley Companies*

Mark's system Mastering Time has been invaluable and has provided something that is almost impossible. It has provided me a format that has given me additional time during the day, allowing me to be more effective and efficient. Thanks Mark, for both the inspiration and guidance.

**BEN LAMON**
*Director of Sales Closet America*

Probably the most important time-management training seminar I have ever attended. I took this seminar early in my career and have used it throughout my professional life in a variety of roles. Mark's system is easy to implement into your daily workflow, and it will increase your productivity without adding more hours to your day.

**TIM BURCH, CR**
*Vice President, Middleburg Office, BOWA*
*Past President/Chairman, NARI Metro DC*
*Lead Project Manager, Extreme Makeover Home Edition, ABC Television*

I was exposed to the system as a new general manager at Case in 2003, and it changed my life. Mark's system allowed me to be more strategic and proactively take control of my day. Additionally, some side benefits included reducing my stress and keeping all my promises both at home and work. I must admit I am guilty of using these techniques on the weekend to make sure the important things get done when it comes to fun.

**STEPHEN SCHOLL, CR, CKBR**

I have been using Mark Richardson's Time Mastery system for over fifteen years and find it invaluable. While it has evolved over time to meet my personal needs and style, the fundamental principles have remained the same. What I love about the system is not just how it provides a mechanism to ensure I stay on track and meet deadlines in a realistic manner, but how it gives me the chance to really think about how I'm using my time and how much time I'm devoting to each "bucket," or area of focus I need to tackle each day. It allows me to think beyond the immediate tasks at hand by also incorporating big-picture goals into my plan.

**MICHELLE DOISCHEN**
*President, Samantha Jordyn Marketing, LLC*

# THE ART OF
# TIME MASTERY

# THE ART OF
# TIME MASTERY

THE **7 STEPS** FOR MASTERING YOUR TIME

## MARK G. RICHARDSON

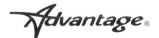

Published by Advantage, Charleston, South Carolina.
Member of Advantage Media Group.

ADVANTAGE is a registered trademark, and the Advantage colophon is a trademark of Advantage Media Group, Inc.

Printed in the United States of America.

10   9   8   7   6   5   4   3   2   1

ISBN: 978-1-64225-080-0
LCCN: 2018962527

Cover and layout design by George Stevens.

This publication is designed to provide accurate and authoritative information in regard to the subject matter covered. It is sold with the understanding that the publisher is not engaged in rendering legal, accounting, or other professional services. If legal advice or other expert assistance is required, the services of a competent professional person should be sought.

Advantage Media Group is proud to be a part of the Tree Neutral® program. Tree Neutral offsets the number of trees consumed in the production and printing of this book by taking proactive steps such as planting trees in direct proportion to the number of trees used to print books. To learn more about Tree Neutral, please visit www.treeneutral.com.

Advantage Media Group is a publisher of business, self-improvement, and professional development books. We help entrepreneurs, business leaders, and professionals share their Stories, Passion, and Knowledge to help others Learn & Grow. Do you have a manuscript or book idea that you would like us to consider for publishing? Please visit advantagefamily.com or call 1.866.775.1696.

*To all those who have made mastering time a priority.*

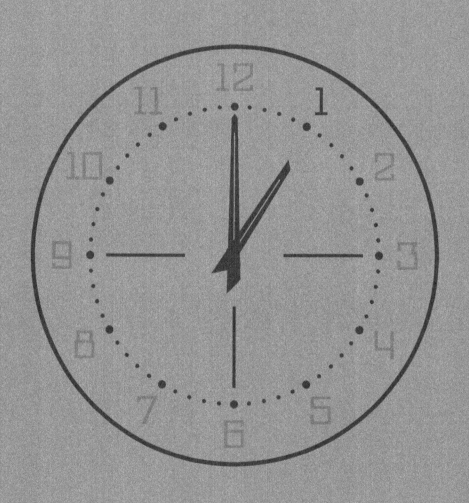

# ACKNOWLEDGMENTS

．．．．．．．．．．．．．．．．．．．．．．．．．．．．．．．．．．．．．．．．．．．．．．．．．．

**W**riting an acknowledgment feels like writing your own obituary. Whether you have written a book or not, an acknowledgement is more about an author's reflections than communication to the reader. Those who know me (very few of you do) know I am very passionate about learning and listening to new ideas and insights. These can come in many forms and from many directions. So I will attempt to acknowledge those who have been important in the time-mastery journey.

I begin with my parents, James and Sheila Richardson, who laid my life's foundation, which is both solid and wide reaching. They created an environment for learning and experimentation and a big safety net to reduce risks.

I also want to acknowledge Thomas Regan, my architecture advisor at Virginia Tech and my first true mentor. Professor Regan taught me how to think through the language of architecture. He pushed me to see the world through multiple lenses. He gave me a methodology that could be translated into many areas of life (including writing).

Next is Fred Case. Fred created a landscape where I could flourish and grow. The results of this growth and accomplishment have allowed me to expand my reach and help others touch greatness.

In addition to this foundation, I want to thank my wife, Margie, and my kids, Jessica, Jamie, and Brett. They are my "why." They keep me grounded and humble. Margie pushes me to excellence when good may have sufficed.

I also want to acknowledge a few advisors who have inspired me to push the teaching of time mastery to the place where I can write this book: first, Bill Baldwin (my first student); then, Tammy Ruffin, Steve Scholl, Rob Patterson, Michelle Doischen, Laurie Griel, Melissa Kennedy, Beth Yuen, Anthony Nardo, Mary Miksch, Sam Imhof, Tim Burch, Bill Millholland, Jeff Miller, Tim Walker, Homa Nowrouzi, Sam Imhof, Keith Vaughn, Shashi Bellamkonda, and Jonathon Katz; and, last but not least, all the others who have consciously or subconsciously given me concepts, ideas, and inspiration.

# TABLE OF CONTENTS

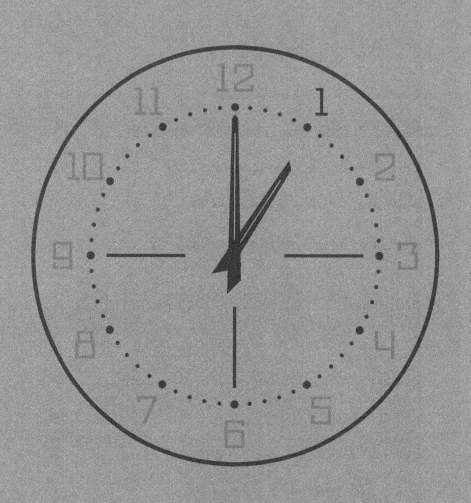

# INTRODUCTION

*"I wasted time, and now doth time waste me."*

**WILLIAM SHAKESPEARE**

T ime. It's a simple concept. Anyone can tell you the time of the day. Or they can tell you the number of hours in a day or days in a week. Time is something we can quantify in a consistent, numerical way. We can measure it and use it to compare. We communicate about time every day. Most people get paid based on the amount of time they work. This is all very straightforward. But if you ask the same people to explain what time *means* to them, the answers vary because even though time is very simple to understand, it is hard to control or master.

I became interested in the subject of time in the late 1980s. I was feeling overwhelmed and stressed by all the balls I was juggling. A friend suggested that I take a time-management course. I found a one-day seminar taught by a University of Maryland professor. The morning was spent discussing time on a very long-term level—ten years and beyond. The professor had us do exercises to visualize what our lives might look like in ten years. After lunch, we began drilling down into the five-year perspective, then one year, then one month. The last hour of the class was spent focusing on planning one single day. It seemed very logical to evaluate time on a macro level and then work our way down to the micro level of daily tasks. I remember coming away that day feeling stimulated intellectually. However, I did not know how to apply what I had learned the next day. Like other failed attempts to improve something, I just went back to my old patterns and routines that did nothing to reduce my stress.

The pain I was experiencing from overwhelm was not going away, and my thirst to do more only made it worse. So I decided to crack the code on my own. Because my background is in architecture and design, I have always found that diagramming and making things visual helped me understand them better. I, like many others, had been making "to-do" lists and had been taught to prioritize and focus on the tougher things first. While these simple techniques made sense, I still felt crappy at the end of the day unless several things were crossed off my list.

Using my architectural thinking process, I decided to approach this daily exercise as if I were designing a project. First, I needed to identify all the "givens" or "ingredients." This is like compiling a "to-do" list. After doing what I call a "brain dump," I could visualize the pieces. I would then try to analyze each item with more detail and estimate the amount of time each activity should take. I would add the total amount of time for all the tasks and would see how that compared to the time available in a day. At first it was difficult to get this to match up, but with practice, I became better at it. I also needed a way to visualize my day. Since I was proficient with timelines and Gantt charts from construction projects, I simply used these same visual tools.

It was a learning process, but I developed a system that began to save minutes here and minutes there—and people began to notice. In 1991, I had a project manager ask me if I could teach him my time-management strategy because he saw the difference in my productivity and wanted to have the same. He began to use my techniques and tools successfully and then told several others in my company how he learned to get his days under control. That led to my giving a time-management seminar for my company. Word about my successful visual techniques spread throughout local and national associations, and I became sort of a go-to speaker on the subject. I became the architectural thinker with the design-based system to take control of your day.

Over the past twenty-five years, I have presented this topic to more than ten thousand people. I would *like* to tell you there are ten thousand users of my techniques, but that would not be true. I will say, however, that most people do look at time a little differently now. Most have a yearning to constantly improve time effectiveness. I can only guess, but I would estimate that 10 to 20 percent of the attendees use these techniques daily and reap benefits such as accomplishing more, feeling less overwhelmed, keeping promises more consistently, and thinking more clearly.

I cannot promise you will buy into or use these techniques, but I can guarantee this process works for most people if they follow it closely. Many people have gone from being frustrated to being in control of their days and thus being more fulfilled.

This book focuses on your time mind-set; gives you the actual tools, tactics, and techniques of time mastery; and helps you create successful habits. So let us begin this time-mastery journey together.

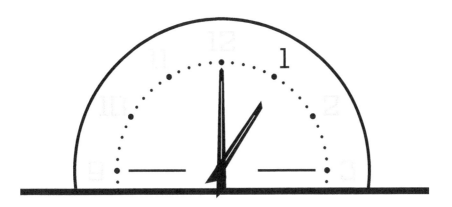

# UNDERSTANDING TIME

*"Time is an illusion."*

ALBERT EINSTEIN

f you want to excel or improve in an activity or discipline, you need to first begin to invest some energy in thinking about it and understanding it better. This understanding not only leads to an opportunity to master it but also to embrace it and enjoy the process.

It is hard to enjoy watching a football game if you don't understand the number of points a team receives when it makes a touchdown. It is also difficult to appreciate this sport if you don't know the basic language the commentator is using to describe different roles on the field.

While you have lived with time all your life there are still some important concepts and themes to understand better, which I present in the following chapters.

## CHAPTER 1

* * * * * * * * * * * * * * * * * * * * * * * * * * * * * * * * * * * * * * *

# EFFICIENT VS. EFFECTIVE

*Every day is a bank account, and time is our currency. No one is rich, no one is poor, and we've got twenty-four hours each.*

CHRISTOPHER RICE

Mastering time involves being both efficient and effective—not just one or the other. When you understand each of these better, you can marry them and see the ideal outcome or balance. Let's begin by looking at some simple definitions of each.

| EFFICIENT | EFFECTIVE |
|---|---|
| *Performing or functioning in a manner that takes the least time and effort.* | *Accomplishing the purpose or producing the intended result.* |

Many people use these words interchangeably, but they really have important differences. I often will look at how someone is doing a task or an activity and ask if it is being done in the least amount of time. I think nobody wants to waste time, so we often judge the success of an activity at least partially by how efficient we are in doing it—the amount of time it took.

Others might judge the success or failure based purely on whether you accomplished the goal.

Let's use a simple example that will illustrate the differences and how you might marry the two.

Bob needs to go to the grocery store on his way home from work to pick up some food for the family dinner. He jots down a quick list as he is sitting at the red light. He parks very close to the entrance (in a loading zone) and leaves his blinkers on. He runs into the store, grabs a handbasket, and quickly throws the items from his list in the basket. He is back in his car in eight minutes, ready to head home. He gets home and, while he got all the items on his list, he had not thought about needing a bottle of wine to go with the meal. He then makes the meal in an efficient manner and is done with the dinner by 7:30 p.m. Was this efficient? Most would say yes. Was it a great meal? Most would say "not really." While it fulfilled his hunger, it was not a memorable dining experience without the wine.

So imagine the scenario this way: Bob arrives at the same store without a list and parks out in the middle of the parking lot. He is not 100 percent sure what he will be buying, so he gets a large shopping cart. He knows he wants to grill something but is not sure what it is. So he begins at one end of the store, seeing if something will inspire him. As he strolls along, he bumps into an old friend he has not seen for six months. They have kids at the same school, so he catches up on the latest news. After about twenty minutes of catching up, he sees the store has some interesting fresh fish. There is a woman buying some, and he asks about the catch of the day. She says she finds this may be one of the best values in the store, shares how she found a recipe online, and describes how she grills this to make it an amazing meal. Bob decides that this really fits the bill and buys some too. Bob proceeds past the wine area and finds that his favorite wine is on sale, so he decides to stock up on a few bottles. After being in the store about forty-five minutes, Bob checks out and heads home.

Bob then dives into preparing the meal with his favored wine. Over dinner he shares his new insights about the school and completes his dinner about nine p.m.

These stories help to illustrate being efficient versus being effective. You could say in the first story Bob is more efficient; but is he more effective? Did he do it?

Not really. If Bob had taken a few minutes to think about the direction the meal might take or asked about other things he could accomplish or buy while he was at the store, he might have had a great meal, picked up a few school insights, and replenished his wine cellar.

In the second scenario, could Bob have done some things to be more efficient? I think you would say the answer is yes. However, with all that he accomplished, was he more effective? I would say yes.

It is important not to see planning as being mechanical or robotic. If Bob had spent five minutes doing a brain-dump list, shortened the conversation with the friend (and set up a time to chat further), and called home to get the grill started, he might have been finished with the whole process by 8:15 p.m. and had a wonderful meal with all the latest intel on the community.

I generally find that—when it comes to basic efficiency and effectiveness on activities and tasks—if I don't know the answers, I like to at least ask questions, such as the following:

1. **Is there another way to do this that might be more efficient or help in accomplishing other interests or goals?**

2. **Is there a way to leverage this activity into accomplishing more than just one task?**

3. **Can I multitask while doing the mundane parts of this activity?**

4. **Is there an opportunity to learn or experience something new?**

5. **How can I also think two or three steps ahead and be better prepared?**

6. **How much time will this take? Is there a way to save five or ten minutes?**

7. **Does this activity or task help me to achieve my medium- or long-term goals?**

By understanding the topic of being efficient versus effective, you will be better at balancing them both. By asking yourself and others questions, you will unleash the greatest computer in existence (your brain) to come up with better ways to do things. As you move along this journey to be more masterful of time, you will find that a higher level of sensitivity is a step toward that goal.

# TIME MYTHS

**Faster is better**. No, *better* is better. This is especially true when it comes to time. I have a friend who always schedules meetings for twenty minutes. His thought process is good, but seven out of ten meetings result in incompleteness or in being rushed. I often find the crown jewels are in the little gaps of time or the little extra breathing room. I recommend setting the amount of time you think you'll need (e.g., twenty minutes) then adding just a little time (say five to ten minutes) for that extra cool idea or interaction.

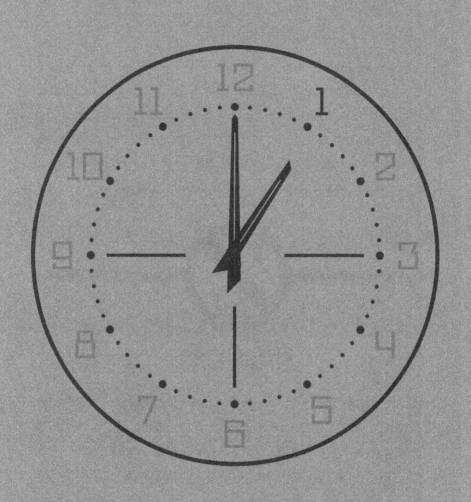

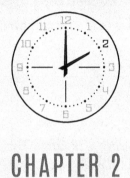

# CHAPTER 2

· · · · · · · · · · · · · · · · · · · · · · · · · · · · · · · · · · · · · · · · · · · · · · · · · · · · · · · ·

# PROACTIVE TIME VS.
# REACTIVE TIME

*Time is the most valuable thing*
*that a man can spend.*

DIOGENES LAËRTIUS

While we are all given the same twenty-four hours in a day, one of the big differences is whether or not we are controlling the *use* of our time.

One way to begin better understanding time is to put our available moments into two separate buckets. The first is the time that we control (what I would call *proactive*). This is the time that goes into deciding what you are going to do along with the amount of time you want or need to devote to doing it. As you will read, the amount of time you decide to commit to something is often the time it takes to actually accomplish the task. It is a choice.

The second bucket is *reactive* time. This is time that you cannot control or that is controlled by others. We all have reactive time; however, the difference between people who are more masterful with time and those not very proficient with it is the percentage of proactive versus reactive time in their day. Understanding each more deeply will allow you to improve.

## PROACTIVE TIME: TIME YOU CONTROL

Examples of proactive time might be the amount of time it takes you to do simple regular tasks like getting ready for work or eating lunch. If you determine that you need thirty minutes to perform a task like this successfully, then you allow the thirty minutes and move on with it. Other proactive time examples could involve a staff or client meeting or a project like writing an outline. You may need to be a little more flexible on what goes into the periods of time allowed, but if you estimate accurately, you should be proactive in that you control the amount of time dedicated to a task.

Another reason that the amount of proactive time is important is that you can *plan* it. You have a choice to spend less or more time to improve effectiveness. You can get creative with proactive time and find ways to reduce it or squeeze more out of it for a better return on your investment.

## Reactive Time: Time That Others Control

We all know what reactive time is. Some common reactive activities include getting caught in a traffic jam or spilling coffee on a shirt and needing to change it. This may seem overly simplistic, but things like this happen throughout any day and we cannot plan for them. Other reactive activities, such as interruptions by clients or team members, throw us off our proactive plan—and are things that we can potentially control better. I have found that there is a basic but big cultural difference between those businesses that have a great deal of reactive activity and those that have much less. While reducing it and controlling it is important, I think allowing for the right amount of reactive dynamic is also where some creative ideas and deeper relationships are built.

As you begin to understand this subject a little more, I suggest you take a quick inventory of your day or week. Such an inventory can be done by asking two simple questions, then taking time to do some analyses to validate your gut.

**Question one:** What percentage of your day or week is "proactive"?

_____

**Question two:** What percentage of your day or week is "reactive"?

_____

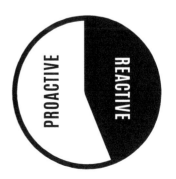

While there is no right or wrong blend, I have found some truisms:

1.  The higher the percentage of proactive time, the better.

2.  People who accomplish more generally have a higher proactive percentage.

3.  Your job or role in a business has some effect on the blend. (e.g., a receptionist has a high percentage of reactive time, while a manager ideally should have a low percentage of reactive time).

4.  If your proactive number is less than 85 percent, you can generally improve it with the right mind-set and techniques.

5.  By following a daily planning system, you can dramatically improve this blend.

The time-mastery system will give you a tool to improve in this area; however, there are three primary sources of reactive time for most people. If you begin to recognize these sources, you can immediately begin to improve and shift some of the reactive time toward being more proactive.

1.  **Your clients:** Reacting to client needs is important for any client-centric organization, but you can develop a win-win dynamic with respect to reducing reactive time. Generally, while they may appreciate your willingness to react, it may not give them the best advice or outcome. While this may seem overly simplistic and general, I think you can adopt the following steps into your world or situation:

a. On Monday morning ask yourself, "Whom would I like to interact with this week? Who might have an issue arise that I will need to address?"

b. With a list of clients or client situations, proactively connect to each with a simple e-mail or text: "John: I know there are a few loose ends on your project that need attention this week. Would you be available on Wednesday at noon (or at 3:00 p.m.) for a twenty-minute catch-up call so I can help with these and any other questions you might have?"

c. As you get answers back, you can lock these times in on your schedule and move them to the proactive-time bucket.

Generally, I find you will get four or five out of ten clients going along with your respectful desire to be proactive. You will get two or three who don't care. Then you will get two or three who won't give up their desire to control you and may actually add to your reactiveness. Over time you will see a 50 to 75 percent improvement, which could change your 50 percent reactive and 50 percent proactive blend to 60/40 or 65/35.

2. **Your team/coworkers:** Being interrupted by your team with a question or an issue that needs your attention can be a big source of reactive time. People who end their day wondering what they got accomplished that day are generally a sponge for this type of reactive time. The question I asked myself many years ago was "Am I really

giving them the respect they deserve when I am interrupted and annoyed?" No. So the following is a process to consider:

a.  When people interrupt you,  ask if you can get back to them at a specific time to address their questions/issues.

b.  If they say okay, make sure you keep your promise.

c.  If they say no, ask them for the specific amount of time they need at that moment (and make them keep the promise).

Of course, there are some fires that need to be addressed immediately. However, out of ten interruptions, at least five will say they can wait; two to three will need addressing immediately; and two to three will vaporize because they came up with solutions themselves. Even a small shift of 5 or 10 percent of your time becoming more proactive can lead to a major shift over time.

3.  **The family:** I think you can use the same methodology with your family; however, try not to be too mechanical or controlling. I am often asked about the difference between the weekday and weekend planning—and the biggest difference is the percentage of reactive time. On weekends, I generally surrender more of my time to my family's control.

The key to this theme is not just about getting the percentage of proactive time higher. It is about reducing the stress that reactiveness causes. It is about neither accomplishing more nor being constantly interrupted. It is about feeling better and more fulfilled at the end of the day. If you can begin to embrace this concept and start practicing some of the techniques, you will find the time-mastery system an easy way to build on your success.

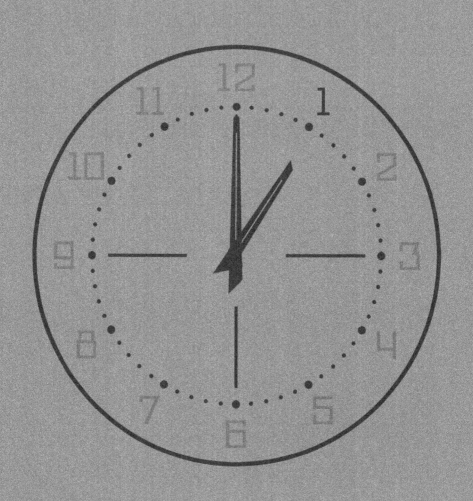

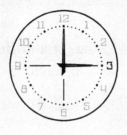

## CHAPTER 3

FINDING THE CADENCE

*There is more to life than simply
increasing its speed.*

Mahatma Gandhi

Success or failure in baking depends upon mixing the right ingredients together. It also depends on "how" the ingredients are mixed and "how long" something is baked in the oven.

While the concept of time may be a little elusive, the more you study the "how," the more masterful you will become. In the coming chapters, we'll talk about ways to make time more meaningful and easier to visualize in the coming chapters. But first, it's important to understand how you use the time you have.

To begin, it's important to understand time *rhythms*. This topic can be analyzed many ways, but let's focus on three particular rhythm questions that are important to mastering time.

1. When is the right time of day to do this?

2. When is the best time of day for my energy and mental state to do this activity?

3. How long should I invest in this activity today?

Most people have times of the day when we are more effective at accomplishing certain activities. Unfortunately we cannot always control when things need to get done, but with the right discipline, we usually can make a big difference in our planning. For a personal example, I find the best time to reflect on goals or long-term ideas and plans is very early in the morning. That is when my mind is strongest, allowing great ideas and thoughts in. It can be a very meditative time. Midmorning is when I usually feel most creative. That is when I schedule time to write, work on talks and podcasts, or move project concepts forward. Midday I am better at focusing on relationships, presentations, and conversations, so I use that time to focus on doing webinars, meetings, and conference calls. The last leg of my day is generally best for busy work or more methodical activities. This is not meant to be robotic, but knowing and understanding these mental cycles or rhythms helps me be more effective.

How does your day break out?

| | Your Cycles in the Day | |
|---|---|---|
| **TIME OF DAY** | **MIND-SET** | **ACTIVITY** |
| *Early Morning* | *Reflective* | *Planning* |
| *Midmorning* | *Creative* | *Projects* |
| *Lunch* | | |
| *Afternoon* | | |
| *Late Afternoon* | *Listening* | *Conversing* |
| *Evening* | | |
| *Late Evening* | | |

Break your day into five to eight parts. For example: early morning, midmorning, lunch, afternoon, late afternoon, evening, and late evening.

Then describe your mind-set and the type of activities you want to accomplish in each portion of your day. For example, very early: meditative/planning—exercise; midmorning: creative thinking—develop new project ideas.

You will use this knowledge to help determine the timing of different activities as you get deeper into the planning system.

# TIME MYTHS

**"There is not enough time for *x*."** This is not true. You may choose not to invest the time, but the amount of time does exist. Generally, I try to get people to think first about the importance of a task and then try to quantify the amount of time for its successful completion. Then you can plan and find the time in the day to do it. I was doing a workshop with a group in California where the manager said he did not have time to take inventory and develop an improvement plan for his seven team members. I said, "Okay, can we do a simple timed exercise?" He agreed.

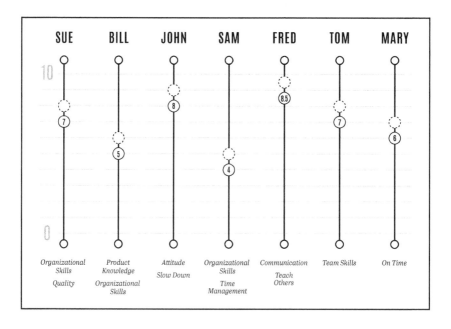

I asked him to give me the names of his seven team members. I wrote down the names on the flip chart. I then asked him to score each one on a zero-to-ten scale on the present overall effectiveness in their job; I added this next to their names. Then I asked him to give me one to three things that each member could do to increase his or her score by one point. He then shared the ideas. Then I stopped the clock.

This process took four minutes. He got my point. (I hope you do too.)

I have found there is almost always enough time for anything we have to do, if we just choose to do it properly. Always try to quantify— then decide how to make it happen.

Another important aspect of time cycle involves *when* is the best portion of the day to accomplish goals or be more effective. If you want to have people focused for a staff meeting, what is the best part of the day for them? If you need to do simple calls, can they be done while you are in your car or in between meetings? I often find "one-on-one" discussions that need a more relaxed dynamic are often best done over lunch or breakfast.

The third time cycle to consider is the length of time to invest into moving a project or task forward. Later, we discuss some basic time-estimating concepts, but this relates more to understanding and unpacking the right things at the right time. For example, you have three weeks to prepare a presentation for a meeting. One approach is to carve out a big chunk of time, knock it out completely, and be ready a week or two early. A better approach might be to break the preparation into parts. Begin with a thirty-minute brainstorm of some ideas for your talk. A couple of days later, share these ideas with a trusted advisor. A few days after that, spend thirty minutes writing a content outline and some key action items. A few days later, dive in and begin to put the parts together in a rough draft. Then you might get some feedback from colleagues. Finally, about four days before the presentation, you will be ready to wrap up a killer presentation. You will have also managed to move the presentation preparation along effectively while still addressing the many other activities in your days and weeks. Moving things too quickly or too slowly is not effective, so it's important to think about the "how" not just the "what."

## JONES PRESENTATION = 6 HRS

*vs.*

## JONES PRESENTATION =

| Day 1 | Brainstorm | 30 minutes |
|-------|------------|------------|
| Day 2 | Discuss Approach | 60 minutes |
| Day 3 | Outline | 30 minutes |
| Day 4 | Draft Presentation | 90 minutes |
| Day 5 | Feedback | 60 minutes |
| Day 6 | Final Presentation | 60 minutes |

This leads to the concept of *cadence*. This is important in sports such as running or cycling. Finding the right cadence can be the difference between winning and losing. I learned this the hard way years ago in a cycling race. As an inexperienced cyclist (but in good shape), I started the race at a very strong pace ahead of the pack. Feeling confident, I thought if I kept up this pace I would have a great race.

About 75 percent of the way to the finish line, I ran out of gas, and I ended up with a very mediocre time. As I became better trained, I began to race based on the right heart-rate cadence. I also began to take on food and fluids at the right time, whether I was hungry or not. Knowing the right racing cadence not only improved the time but also allowed me to enjoy the ride more.

This theme holds true in mastering not only your time but also how you communicate time to others. A question I often ask myself or others is "Is this time allowed aggressive but realistic?" *Aggressive* means not being lazy or slow. *Realistic* means it can be accomplished in the amount of time available for completion without sacrificing other important tasks. If you consistently ask this question, you will get better at both hitting the time allowed and communicating and having others fit into your timetable. A simple metaphor that visually illustrates this theme is a rubber band. If it is limp—**not aggressive**—it does you no good. If you pull it too far—**too aggressive**—it will snap. If you give it the right tension—**aggressive but realistic**—it functions very effectively.

## AGGRESSIVE BUT REALISTIC | *The Rubber Band*

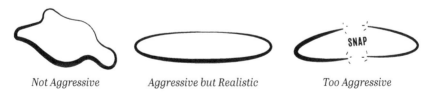

*Not Aggressive*  *Aggressive but Realistic*  *Too Aggressive*

Time mastery, in some ways, is like putting together pieces of a jigsaw puzzle, and cadence is one of the most important pieces. If you can focus on when is the best time and question how long something should realistically take, you will be much closer to being able to see the big picture.

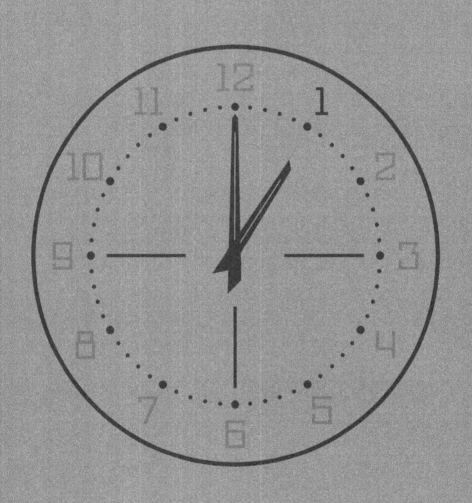

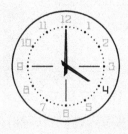

# CHAPTER 4

· · · · · · · · · · · · · · · · · · · · · · · · · · · · · · · · · · · · · · · · · · · · ·

# SAGE THOUGHTS ON TIME

As I try to get my head around any topic or subject, I often find it helpful to seek out what other thought leaders have said about it. Generally, if something is said in an interesting, clever, or unique way it helps you think about a subject differently and gain some additional insights.

Here are quotes about the subject of time and some of my takeaways.

*Time has no meaning in itself unless*
*we choose to give it significance.*

LEO BUSCAGLIA

By putting a spotlight on time, you elevate its importance or give it significance. You also will understand it better and can find ways to leverage it better. It is a choice.

*A man who dares to waste one hour of time has not discovered the value of life.*

CHARLES DARWIN

Well, we have all wasted time but those who waste less time generally value time more.

*Time is money.*

BENJAMIN FRANKLIN

Is time really money? Not really. Is there value in time? Sure. What I like about this simple quote is that if we translate time into something else, we learn to appreciate it more. In a later chapter I take you through an exercise to translate time into meaningful activities. After you do that, you will look at time (or wasting time) very differently.

## *Don't try to do tomorrow's work today.*

### FLORENCE NIGHTINGALE

It's important to know where you are heading, but if you don't put today's foot forward you will never get there. It is tough to stay in the moment, but with the right mind-set, the right system, and the right practice you will get there.

## *Time is what we want most but what we use worst.*

### WILLIAM PENN

We all have said, "If I only had time I would *x*." Or, "Where did the time go?" As I study the people who say these things the least, I find they are usually people who are masterful in understanding their time.

## *Work expands so as to fill the time available for its completion.*

### CYRIL NORTHCOTE PARKINSON

While it is important to not feel pressure to complete everything quickly, we tend to use all the time made available to complete a task. For example, if I go to the grocery store to pick up ingredients for a meal and I do not have time constraints, I will probably wander around the store while grabbing those ten ingredients. I might also say hello and chat with an old friend. I might even pick up a few more things while I am there. This task now takes about forty to fifty minutes to accomplish. On the other hand, if I give myself only twenty minutes to get the ten items, I will most likely avoid distractions and accomplish the same goal. Is the first way more relaxed? Maybe. But it took an extra twenty minutes. If I asked you what an additional twenty minutes each day would represent over the course of a year, you would be shocked. Would you trade adding a daily process to save you twenty minutes a day or 120 hours in a year? Most would say yes.

## *Fail to plan, then plan to fail.*

### BENJAMIN FRANKLIN

Most of us have some level of planning skills in both our personal and professional lives. These plans are generally a process we have been taught and have practiced. Some plans are simple, like planning a meal. Some are more complex, like planning a conference or designing a building. It is not very efficient to reinvent the wheel every time we tackle a meal or a project, so we follow a process. Ironically, we often don't have a written plan to follow and make the best decisions. The daily process and techniques you will learn follow this theme: if you can just invest twenty to thirty minutes a day, you will have a plan that will give you more control and clarity to accomplish your goals.

## *Plan your work and work your plan.*

### UNKNOWN

As noted, having a plan is important. But a daily plan (not just any plan) is critical to your success. Many years ago I heard an interview with a very successful man by the name of Mark McCormack. He was successful in business and his personal life. McCormack was a believer in daily plans. He said he spent about ninety minutes every day planning that day. He was methodical about his process and would not launch his day until the plan was complete and fine-tuned. The time-mastery process in this book provides a methodology to successfully design your day. Most will not spend ninety minutes, so it is designed to be done in twenty to thirty minutes. For the system to work, it must be done daily before you start your day. Then work your plan!

> *Yesterday is gone. Tomorrow has not yet come. We have only today. Let us begin.*

> MOTHER TERESA

While we have the complexity to reflect on the past and look to the future, this simple quote reminds us to live in the moment. It is about focusing intensely on today and then seeing the benefits of that success to build on tomorrow. The time-mastery system follows this simple quote to the tee.

> *Success is a verb.*

> DAN KENNEDY

Success is not a noun (even though most see it as a noun). When you realize that success comes from what you do, not what was done, you can control and master it. Just think, "Make it happen."

There are many other quotes or adages about time/success and inaction that speak for themselves:

*The road to hell is paved with good intentions.*

**PROVERB**

*Practice makes perfect.*

**UNKNOWN**

*How did it get so late so soon?*

**DR. SEUSS**

*Time is the longest distance between two places.*

**TENNESSEE WILLIAMS**

*They always say time changes things, but you actually have to change them yourself.*

**ANDY WARHOL**

These quotes and adages are like pieces of a jigsaw puzzle. They all fit together in an interesting way. If you look at just one piece you have a partial impression. But if you look at many of them joined together you gain an understanding and insight that is much more complete.

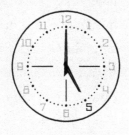

## CHAPTER 5

...................................................

# HOW TIME HAS CHANGED

*Change or become irrelevant.*

CHRIS EDELEN

A friend of mine won a major business award several years ago. In his acceptance speech he said, "If a business is not changing, it will become irrelevant." As I reflected on his words that day, I realized that irrelevance was the worst thing that could happen to a business (or a person). Just maintaining the status quo is not even an option anymore. Embracing how we look at time and how we control it is critical to constantly improving and remaining successful.

When I think about that speech today, it seems so much more relevant. Why is that—has time changed? For thousands of years, humans have recognized twenty-four hours in a day and seven days in a week. So the answer must be no, right?

Like many questions, though, you need to not only look at the "what" but also the "how." When we do, we see that time has changed in a number of ways even in our lifetimes, especially due to changes in technology.

# TIME MYTHS

**If I could sleep less, I could accomplish more.** This was a misconception I had many years ago. I even made it a goal to sleep less. As I get older and wiser, I understand the value of sleep and rest more and more. Study after study has proven that sleep is not only about recharging, but it is also about subconsciously addressing important issues. It is also about buying time to make better decisions. The adage "sleep on it" is important for many reasons. I just encourage a little more proactivity with this subject. Generally, if you're really not sure of the best course, it is better to sleep on it. You can write down an item that you want to sleep on and put it next to your bed, and you will be amazed what the outcome can be.

## HOW TIME HAS CHANGED

| 20 YEARS AGO | | TODAY |
|---|---|---|
| TECHNOLOGY OPTIONAL | ⮕ | DEPENDENT ON TECHNOLOGY |
| TIME BUILT VALUE | ⮕ | TIME IS NOT ON YOUR SIDE |
| "FREE TIME" | ⮕ | TIME IS NOT "FREE" |
| RETURN CALLS NEXT DAY | ⮕ | RETURN CALLS THAT HOUR |
| "OFFICE HOURS" | ⮕ | 24/7 |
| 24 HOURS IN A DAY | ⮕ | 24 HOURS IN A DAY |

# TECHNOLOGY

For years, I have been telling the audiences at workshops and speaking events, "Technology will revolutionize business." I've recently adjusted this a little. Now I say, "Technology has revolutionized *everything*. We are living the future." Whether you embrace this technological wave or not, our real-time relationship with information has drastically changed how we manage our time. Today, technology is not an option; it is both an expectation and dependence.

# BUILDING VALUE WITH TIME

In the late 1980s, I told prospective clients that I would get back to them with design concepts in seven to fourteen days. This allowed us to organize our own workflow, and it also created a perception of value regarding the level of attention the project was getting—one to two weeks felt like a lot of value compared to the one to two days it takes now to do the same thing. Today, however, you win or lose projects by time. Speed sells. Conversion rates increase by the speed at which you can deliver. This happens in our personal lives too. Years ago, a restaurant's quality was often measured by how long you needed to wait to book a table reservation. Today, you pop in or call ahead for a restaurant and if they cannot seat you in a few minutes, most people move on to the next one. Scheduling a service appointment works the same way now: speed of service has become as important to many people as quality and price. While we often see value in the amount of time things take, time really is not on your side like it was years ago.

# FREE TIME

The concept of "free time" has changed drastically too. In the late 1990s, many people divided their time into three parts: work, family, and free time. You would ask new friends or even business interviewees what they did in their "free time." Today this language is not very common. Why? I believe it is because the voids or spare moments of non-work time have been filled with other activities, including more work. We are involved and have access to so many more things that the concept of "free time" has changed. Today, we talk about finding balance in our lives, but time is not a void that needs to be filled. If anything, for most people, the work hours aren't where the cup runneth over the most—it's the minutes when we are not working that are overflowing the most. Time is not *free*.

## RETURNING CALLS

In the late eighties, my receptionist would tell clients that I would call them back within three business days. Then I changed the policy to always return calls within twenty-four hours; at the time, I thought this was a game changer for a client experience. Today, people expect you to return a call or an e-mail or a text *within one hour*. If it takes longer, many people instantly start wondering "Did they get my message?" "Should I be concerned?" "Should I move on and call someone else?" Now, you may not agree with this expectation, but if you can adopt this speed thinking, it can be very meaningful in business and in personal relationships. Think about how you feel if someone does not get back to you quickly.

## OFFICE HOURS

In the early nineties, I treated most of my professional relationships like I would accountants or contractors. I would always ask, "What are your office hours?" With so many ways to reach people and our increased expectations about a quick reply, the question is now more open-ended: "When is the best time to reach you?"

Today, I sometimes get e-mails from my accountants or my editor as early as 5:00 a.m. or as late as 10:00 p.m. I would like to think this is about the importance of their relationship with me, but it is likely more about society's changing expectations about time. I am not proposing that you are "on" 24/7, but I think you would agree this is an example of how things have changed.

We can go on and on comparing things now versus then. Some elements of these changes are good—I like watching a season of my favorite television show without watching an advertisement, conducting conference calls from my car as I drive, or having basic supplies shipped in a day right to my front door. Other changes have only managed to add too many choices and additional stress for a lot of people. There have been many studies to validate the effects of the proliferation of choices and changing expectations. Many businesses have created value propositions primarily focused on speed (e.g., one-hour dry cleaning, one-day bath remodeling, one-day delivery, etc.). We often pay more for speed whether we need it or not.

While I think we can all acknowledge these changes, the difference in being successful is how we individually embrace these changes and how we become masters of time. We'll explore the "how"—the time-mastery system itself—in the second part of this book.

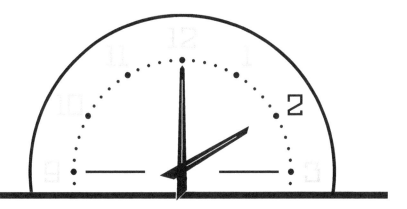

# THE SEVEN STEPS TO MASTERING TIME

*A good plan is like a road map; it
shows the destination and usually
marks the best way to get there.*

H. STANLEY JUDD

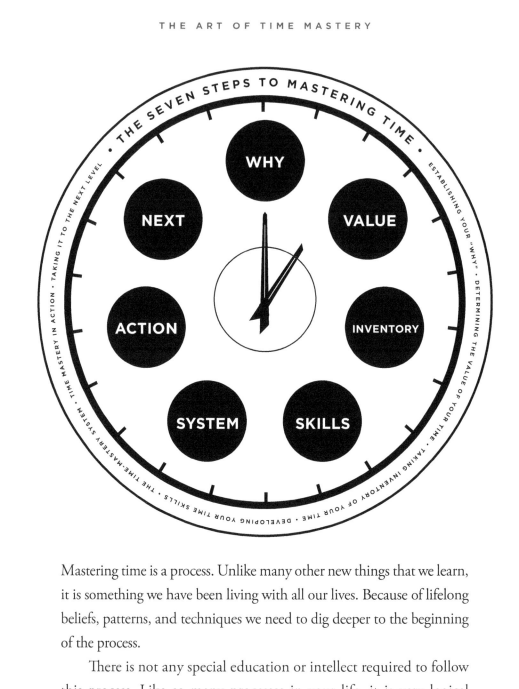

THE SEVEN STEPS TO MASTERING TIME · ESTABLISHING YOUR "WHY" · DETERMINING THE VALUE OF YOUR TIME · TAKING INVENTORY OF YOUR TIME · DEVELOPING YOUR TIME SKILLS · THE TIME-MASTERY SYSTEM · TIME MASTERY IN ACTION · TAKING IT TO THE NEXT LEVEL

WHY
NEXT
VALUE
ACTION
INVENTORY
SYSTEM
SKILLS

Mastering time is a process. Unlike many other new things that we learn, it is something we have been living with all our lives. Because of lifelong beliefs, patterns, and techniques we need to dig deeper to the beginning of the process.

There is not any special education or intellect required to follow this process. Like so many processes in your life, it is very logical and sensible. I have chosen the seven steps I believe are required for this journey. While I do not want you to skip any steps, I would not discourage you from adding a step or two if you think it will help you accomplish your goal of time mastery. While moving along this path, I strongly encourage discipline and focus. Many who attend my seminars fail due to falling off the process. By blocking out thirty minutes each day to do this process, you will not only fully understand it but also understand what is required to see success. Don't hesitate to use my other tools (recordings/webinars/visuals) to help deepen your understanding.

## STEP 1

# ESTABLISHING YOUR "WHY"

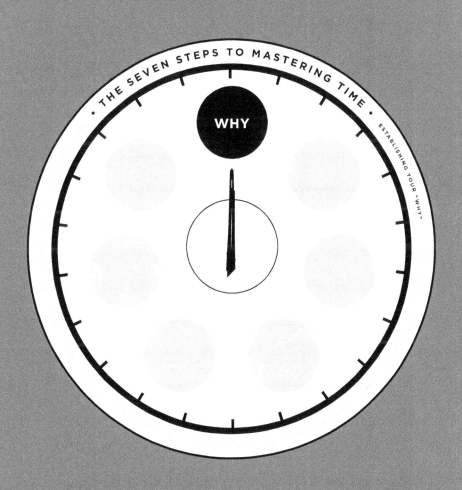

One of the most important questions people should ask themselves is "Why?" By asking this with almost any subject you gain both clarity and motivation.

For example, if you think you want to lose fifteen pounds, you probably have a good reason or two—but do you have enough reasons to actually go through the pain and inconvenience of making it happen? If you begin to list the reasons why you want to lose weight, you might find a pretty long list (including stamina, feeling better, cost of food, health, vanity, cost of health care, save on buying new clothes, pride, positive attitude, etc.).

This same methodology is true when it come to the subject of mastering time. When you begin to brainstorm a list, it is not only very motivating but it also begins to paint a picture as to the strategies and tactics you might want to focus on to master this topic.

So let's begin with making a list.

**"Why is mastering your time important to you?"**

1. _____

2. _____

3. _____

4. _____

5. _____

6. _____

7. _____

## WHY IS MASTERING TIME IMPORTANT?

Over the years, I have asked audiences why taking control of their day would be important to them. Here are the most common seven reasons:

1. **Reduces stress.** Most people today are pretty stressed out. This stress is unhealthy on so many levels. If you have more control over your time, you will find that stress levels will go down.

2. **Allows you to accomplish more.** While this may not be your biggest motivation, accomplishing more is certainly nice. This could include staying connected to old friends or family or giving back to the community. Accomplishing more could mean doing a better job at any activity or task or making more money to invest. The bottom line is, if you have more mastery over your time, then there may be a little extra time in the tank for you to accomplish more.

3. **Allows you to think more clearly.** You are faced with many decisions every day. One characteristic of the most successful people is that they make fewer mistakes. Mistakes can be a product of not thinking things through, considering all the variables, and mapping out all the unintended consequences. By mastering your time, you can build in time to think more clearly too.

4. **Allows you to keep promises.** How do you feel when you don't keep your promises? They may be big or very small promises. Can others always count on you to come through 100 percent of the time with what you say you will do? While none of us are perfect, one byproduct of

mastering your time is keeping promises. As you reflect on people who keep or exceed their promises, you will find they are not only respected—but also quite successful.

5.  **Allows you to focus on medium- and long-term goals.** Most people who struggle with time management spend almost all their time focusing on today or this week. They are reacting and putting out fires just to keep them from spreading. If you are spending most of your time only on the short term, you are compromising the longer vision and direction. Think about driving a car. Drivers who are enjoying the driving experience keep an eye on the immediate car and road around them, but they also appreciate the surrounding landscape and know where they are heading by looking out to the horizon to anticipate the weather or traffic ahead. This metaphor is relevant when you think about your time. By having control and mastery, you give yourself the license to adjust your focus, short, medium, and long term (and better enjoy the ride).

6.  **Reduces overwhelm.** Overwhelm is a feeling that we all have experienced. It is not a good feeling. It causes stress, creates ineffectiveness, and makes us behave with others in an inappropriate manner. As I have studied this subject, I've discovered that it is quantifiable. Overwhelm is created by the proliferation of activities and variables. If you think about overwhelm like a juggler, you can start to understand it better. An amateur juggler can juggle three balls fairly easily. If you add a fourth or a fifth, he or she needs to concentrate more on keeping them in the air. If you add two more balls, then they all fall on the floor

and the juggler gives up in frustration. If you can think of activities that way, it helps in comprehending this theme. If you have only one or two tasks or activities to do, it is pretty easy not to feel overwhelmed. If you then add one or two more, or if you are interrupted by others adding more variables, then overwhelm begins to set in. By mastering your time and controlling the reactive time activities you will reduce overwhelm. (More to come on this.)

7. **Allows you to sleep better at night.** Some people may naturally not be very good sleepers. Most, however, lose sleep because of their environment. This environment could be noise or what you ate the day before. However, as I study this subject, I find that a high percentage of sleep loss is due to things that are whirling around in your head. It could be questions that need to be addressed or stress from deadlines. It also could be that you are trying to think through and organize activities for the next day. By mastering time you will give yourself the permission to shut down. You will be able to better focus in an organized way the next morning. All this allows you to get a better night's sleep.

## KNOW YOUR WHY

There may be several other specific reasons why it would be great to master time. By keeping this why list top of mind, you will have the clarity and mastery to invest the time to get better at controlling time.

When you add all these up, the bottom line is you feel better and more fulfilled.

# TIME MYTHS

**I need to just get out of bed and dive into my day.** I used to think this way. Now I try to stay in bed a little longer after I wake up. It may be fifteen or twenty minutes, but in that amount of time I can let the wave of the day begin to move though me. I can begin to visualize the day. I generally begin to feel the priorities or the positive or negative stress of the pace of the day that will need to be addressed in my plan. I now force myself to stay in bed for this amount of time. After I get out of bed, I find getting ready in the morning to be a more integral part of my planning process. While I brush my teeth or shave, I begin to filter the important questions that will influence my planning exercise. I also have the license to really stretch and think in longer-term intervals that may add a few actions to inch along. This reflective time after waking up is very important to creating a good road map for the day.

# DETERMINING THE VALUE OF YOUR TIME

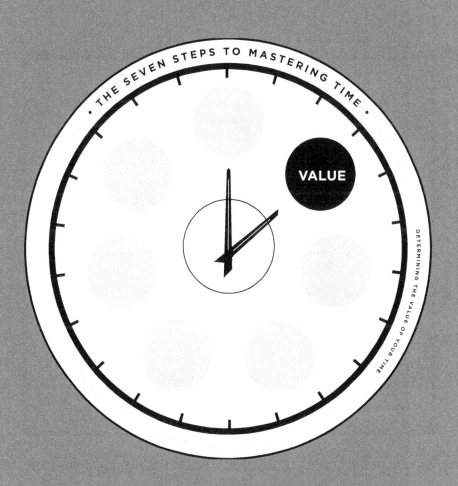

THE SEVEN STEPS TO MASTERING TIME

VALUE

DETERMINING THE VALUE OF YOUR TIME

As we discussed earlier, time is pretty elusive. We all have it, but we cannot see it. We can't touch it. We can't feel it. Time is the difference between winning and losing. Time affects whether we are poor or wealthy. Time is very important.

While I cannot sprinkle magic dust on it so you can literally see it, I can begin to give you ways and techniques to make it more meaningful and help you see its value.

One technique I use for audiences in workshops is to have them list different *amounts* of time. Then we try to attach an activity that is meaningful to them that can be done in that amount of time.

For example:

| | |
|---|---|
| | *Fifteen minutes might mean a short walk with your dog, getting ready for work in the morning, or stopping and grabbing a Starbucks coffee on the way in to work.* |
| | *One hour might mean an exercise class or watching your favorite TV show.* |
| | *Three hours might be a flight from DC to Denver or a drive to the beach.* |
| | *Eight hours might mean building a small deck, a day of work, or Thanksgiving Day with the family.* |

What do these time intervals mean to you?:

| 15 MIN. | |
|---|---|
| 1 HOUR | |
| 3 HOURS | |
| 8 HOURS | |
| 24 HOURS | |

It is important that you find what resonates personally for you for each of these time frames. Then, as you engage in activities that require the same amount of time, (e.g., 1 hour = a staff meeting or a nice dinner with a friend) you begin to require and get the best use and value from your precious time.

By drilling into this deeper, you also push the envelope on what you can accomplish in a short amount of time.

For example, I was curious about how long it took me in the morning to prepare and make a pot of coffee. So I timed it. Initially it took about three minutes. Over time, I began to adjust the steps to be more efficient (and equally effective) and got the process down to one minute and a half. Now if you multiply this time out, I was able to save 9.1 hours in a year. Now what is the value and meaning of 9.1 hours? What can I do with 9.1 hours in a year? If it is billable time, then that is about $2,500. With $2,500 I can buy ten tickets for my wife and me to the Washington Nationals.

This is a simple (and maybe a little obsessive) example; but try to make the value of time more meaningful.

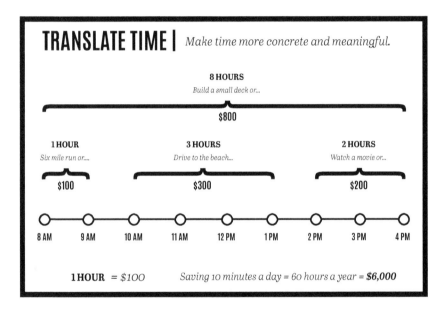

**TRANSLATE TIME |** *Make time more concrete and meaningful.*

**8 HOURS**
*Build a small deck or...*

$800

**1 HOUR**
*Six mile run or...*

$100

**3 HOURS**
*Drive to the beach...*

$300

**2 HOURS**
*Watch a movie or...*

$200

8 AM  9 AM  10 AM  11 AM  12 PM  1 PM  2 PM  3 PM  4 PM

**1 HOUR** = $100      *Saving 10 minutes a day = 60 hours a year = **$6,000***

The key is first to really see the value of each minute. Then look at things you can do to improve these simple activities; and try to celebrate and use the windfall of the time savings in a positive way.

While this step is more of an awareness exercise, you will begin to look at and put more value in the time spent.

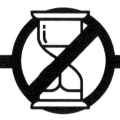

# TIME MYTHS

**Free time. Time is not free; stop using this phrase.** If you begin to realize that you are generally just making a choice on how you invest your time—rather than not planning it—you will see time differently. As you become more proficient at measuring the value of time and comparing activities and the amounts of time they will take, you will stop using the term "free time." I like to blend and leverage professional and personal activities where you can get a lot more done with less stress.

# TAKING INVENTORY OF YOUR TIME

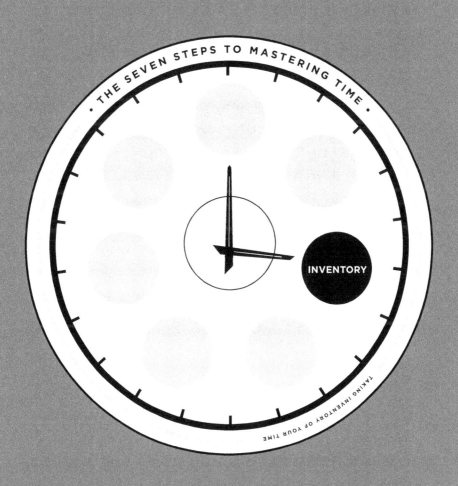

# TIME MYTHS

**I don't have time to exercise.** Exercise might be one of the better things to do not only for your health but also to sharpen your time skills. If you have a limited amount of time, then begin with fifteen minutes a day. I asked a fitness expert, "If I only had fifteen minutes to exercise, what would you recommend?" He said, "Seven minutes of intense cardio, seven minutes of weights (or weight-bearing exercises), and one minute of stretching. I tried it, and really felt as though I'd had a real workout. Needless to say, I would encourage investing more than fifteen minutes, but if that is all you have at first, then start there. Another benefit of the exercise is that it gets the blood flowing in your brain to think more clearly and plan more effectively. My doctor explains how the nerve connections fire up when you exercise and you can supercharge the speed of your thoughts. So begin to think about exercising as a time-mastery tool and you will find the time to make working out a priority.

When you decide to improve on an aspect of your life, whether it's your health, relationships, or sports, it is important to take inventory of where you are now. For example, if you want to lose weight, you might want to evaluate your present caloric intake, the amount of exercise you get each week, and even the daily cycles and structure of your meals. When it comes to taking inventory of time, it may not be quite as tangible or obvious as your weight, but it is equally important and may even be more insightful.

Here are some ways to categorize time to help with your inventory:

1. Proactive time versus reactive time (see the earlier chapter dedicated to this): this is an important exercise to understand and it provides specific tips to set the stage for overall time mastery.

    a. Take a look at your calendar for the last few weeks and reflect on the amount of time you controlled versus reacted to.

    b. Think about an eight- or ten-hour day and the total number of hours that might fall into each bucket.

    c. Some days won't be typical, but try to get an average of a week or two. For example, if on Thursday you were in several meetings all day, then it probably was a high percentage of proactive time versus another day when you were putting out fires. If you average them together, it might give you 50 percent proactive and 50 percent reactive.

    As noted in the earlier chapter this is a foundational element, in that you first need to understand it, then take inventory, then commit to improving it if you ever want to master time.

2. Your other time blends (or time-portfolio blend).

    a. **Short-, medium-, long-term time:** While the ideal blend of time may vary depending upon your role in a business and where you are in your life, we all have the three levels of time. When you feel overwhelmed for an extended period, it is often from spending too much of your focus on short-term efforts only. It is like driving a car and only staring at the hood or just in front of you. It can be exhausting and not as productive.

Determine how much time you are spending on each interval of time. The three levels are defined as short term (this week), medium term (one to two months), and long term (two months or longer). They are sort of like micro versus wide-angle camera lenses. You can do a gut check based on the percentage of time you feel you spend on each, or you can drill deeply into the number of hours per week for each. After you take inventory of your present situation, begin to think about what would be ideal.

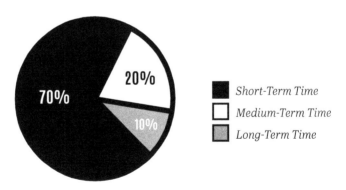

70%

20%

10%

■ Short-Term Time
□ Medium-Term Time
▨ Long-Term Time

# TIME SPENT ON INTERVAL EFFORTS: IDEAL WEEKLY BREAKDOWN

There are instances that require you to focus primarily on short-term time, such as moving a critical project through or putting a major fire out. However, in more normal cases, there should be an ideal blend. For most people, the ideal blend is about 70 to 75 percent short term, 15 to 20 percent medium term, and 10 to 15 percent long term.

b. **The diversity blend of activities in your week:** Another blend to evaluate is the percentage of time spent on the different types of activities in your week. By understanding this, you can begin to adjust it to be more effective and you can look for efficiencies in each. I generally recommend coming up with five to seven categories of activities in your week. For example: (1) meetings, (2) projects, (3) communications, (4) administration, (5) client interactions, (6) reactive time, (7) travel. Everyone has different categories, so don't let identifying the categories paralyze you. After you do this analysis a few times, fine-tune the categories to be more personally accurate and meaningful. Attach the number of hours or percentage of your time to each category in an average week. Set this analysis down and consider what your ideal percentage or blend should be. Compare the two and think about the gaps that need improvement.

| | BLEND OF ACTIVITIES (50-HOUR WEEK) | | |
|---|---|---|---|
| | HOURS PER WEEK | % | IDEAL |
| Meetings | 10 | | 8 |
| Projects | 9 | | 13 |
| Communication | 3 | | 3 |
| Administrative | 4 | | 3 |
| Client Interactions | 6 | | 10 |
| Reactive Time | 10 | | 5 |
| Travel | 8 | | 8 |

c. **Work/family/you blend:** Another blend to evaluate is the blend of time you spend working versus with your family versus on yourself. Again, as I find when I am coaching business leaders, by asking this question you will find if you are in balance. You might be feeling resentful or frustrated. By taking inventory, you might reveal why. As an example, I did a deep dive into my travel schedule last year and discovered that the eighteen additional trips that had been added to my schedule took about 150 hours away from the time I had committed to myself and my writing. Thus, I was neither fulfilling my obligation to my publisher nor to myself. It was through this inventory that I could see, understand, and quantify the problem.

Your blend is a choice you control. I am not here to tell you what your blend should be. A good friend of mine believes you should only work as much as you need to fulfill your family's financial needs. Another friend finds his work a source of learning and cannot get enough of it. Finding your personal balance or blend is what is important.

How do you measure up to others? Do they think your balance is good, or can it be improved? This may be more subjective, but it will add to your understanding of the subject and give you clarity and motivation to adjust and change.

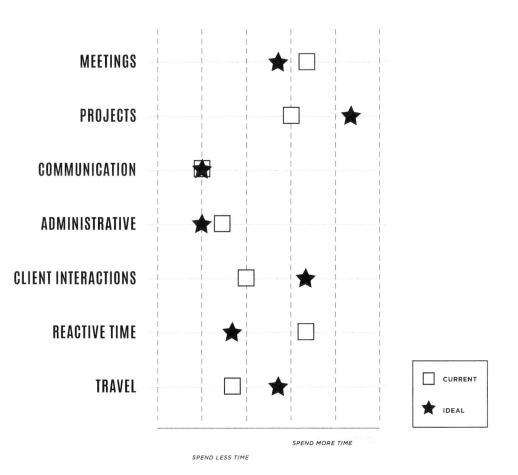

Try to find the gaps between actual time and ideal time. This is where you will see goals and ways to improve. For example, if you find your reactive time is above 20 percent, then begin to apply some of the tips that were discussed in the earlier chapter. If you are spending very little time on long term, begin by blocking out a sixty-minute appointment with yourself each week (just like you would with a client or team member) to plan for the long term. If your health is slipping because you don't have time to exercise, invest the time by planning and scheduling it.

We are all seeking balance. We all want to invest the right amount of ourselves in the right things at the right times. If you want to master your time, you must know where you stand now. Spend some time and have fun taking inventory. You will probably be surprised at the gems of time you might discover.

## TOP-TEN TIME WASTERS

*Time you enjoy wasting is not wasted time.*

BERTRAND RUSSELL

As you become more conscious of time and make it a priority, you begin to realize that much of the success comes from three things:

1.  Understanding it

2.  Adopting and acting on new techniques and approaches

3.  **Not doing things that waste time.**

When you quantify what makes the biggest difference, it might be less about adding new approaches and more about *eliminating* things.

Recently I heard someone draw a parallel of wasted time to a leaky faucet. If you don't fix the leak, over time you will have a big water bill. When we have a major pipe burst, we fix it quickly. However, the amount of waste or size of the water bill can be much greater with the drips than the burst. If you reduce or stop the drips of wasted time, it can have a huge benefit to achieve the success you yearn for. Remember, just ten minutes of drips of time per day equals sixty hours in a year.

The following are common time wasters. Maybe not all of them apply to you. Perhaps there are a few that you can tweak and you will see marginal improvement. Then again, there may be one or two that really hit a nerve and will make a big difference for you.

 1.  **Talking without listening.** Listening is a choice. Listening is a muscle that needs conditioning. Not listening wastes time. Think about people you know who are guilty of this. At times, everyone is guilty of talking too much—but at least try to recognize when you are doing this and practice "active listening." If you are focused on asking questions, then shutting up, you can get through a ten-minute conversation in five minutes—with a better outcome and clearer understanding of next steps.

 2.  **Not writing things down.** I know this sounds a little patronizing, but writing things down is not only about documenting; it is also about giving yourself permission not to have to remember. When you do not have to remember, you can

be in the moment. When you are in the moment, you listen and have more synergistic creative thoughts. If you don't write things down, you not only waste time trying to remember or needing someone to repeat, but also you are not opening up your brain to think ahead about your next move effectively.

3.    **Interruptions.** Interruptions exist for everyone. They exist at many levels (the power goes off in the office or you get a request for help from a team member). The reason these interruptions are a big time waster (and can be improved upon) is that we do not know how to react or deal with them. In the chapter about proactive and reactive time, I address this. If you can begin to control three or four of the ten interruptions a day, you will save hundreds of hours per year.

4.    **Not leveraging your time.** You are a very complex being. You can accomplish more than one thing at a time. I believe one time waster is doing simple required tasks and not leveraging that time to accomplish other things too. Some obvious examples are (1) driving, (2) exercising, and (3) eating. There are many others like walking the dog or waiting for a doctor's appointment or even watching TV. Now, you may choose not to leverage these, but you must at least acknowledge that there is an opportunity—by just doing a few additional simple tasks—to not waste time. For example, I make a list of calls so I can easily march through them on a twenty- or thirty-minute drive. Or I

use my exercise time to read a draft of a column or brainstorm a podcast topic. Multitasking is an opportunity to leverage time. If you look carefully at your day, you can find creative ways to leverage your time. It's a mistake not to use this time.

 5. **Being late.** Being late is not only disrespectful; it also can waste your time. If you are late for a dinner reservation, you may lose your table. If you're late for a meeting, not only do you waste other people's time, the flow of the agenda may need to be repeated or shortened and rendered ineffective. Life would be so much better if you could count on everyone being on time. Successful people are not late!

# TIME MYTHS

**It is okay to be a few minutes late.** Wrong. Masters of time are on time. They understand that being late not only is unprofessional but also can snowball and throw off many minutes in the day that they can never get back. There is an amusing quote that many Americans believe: "late + excuse = on time."

6. **Allowing others to control you.** People who control generally don't waste their time. Finding a balance is important in normal relationships, but try to be the one controlling, and you will not waste time. This is not about who is the boss. I have known many executive assistants who manage up as well as down, and they don't waste time.

 7. **Being too slow or too fast.** Finding the right amount of time and the right cadence is important. In the absence of this, you can waste time. If you give yourself thirty minutes to pick up milk and cheese at the store when you could do it in fifteen minutes, your internal cycle will use more of the time and waste a few minutes. The flipside is also true in that, if you only give yourself ten minutes, you might make a mistake or need to go back for another trip. As you begin to master time you also master the cadence and pace to do things right with the right amount of time.

 8. **Not saying no (gracefully).** Most of us are pleasers who want to help others. Most of us believe when we are asked to help, saying yes is the best answer. I am not encouraging you to be unkind or unhelpful. I do believe, though, that always saying yes is a time waster for you. As you begin to quantify this, do some simple math. If with ten requests (personal or professional) you can just say no (or at least "not now") to two or three of the interruptions you are most reluctant to do, and with two or three ask if you can respond back in

an hour or two, you will get a big dividend in return. The key is to be graceful, kind, and effective.

 9. **Doing things that you should not do.** If there are ten to fifteen things in the day that you do, I would be willing to bet that a few of those could have been eliminated—and that you would look back at them and say, "That was a waste of time." The best way to address this is to think more deeply before you commit to something. A few questions you might run through your filter are: (a) Do I really need to do this? (b) Is there a better way to accomplish it? (c) What is the worst thing that will happen if I don't do it? Again, the point is to not waste time. If you can eliminate a few of these ten to fifteen things, then you can use the time more effectively (even if it is just taking a nap).

 10. **Not having a plan.** Think about jumping in the car and needing to make five stops but not planning your route beforehand. Or what if you are preparing a special meal for friends and you go to the grocery store without making a shopping list? You wouldn't dive into a remodeling project without preparing a sketch or a material list. The same is true as you move through your day. By not having a plan, you are sure to waste time. You will make mistakes. You will need to redo things. You will not be able to see some of the efficiencies in front of you.

What are your time wasters? List your top ten.

_____

_____

_____

_____

_____

_____

_____

_____

_____

_____

Use these strategies as a checklist. Rate yourself from zero to ten on each of these time wasters. Focus on improving one or two where you have the lowest scores. If you do, you will receive a priceless gift—time. This gift did not cost you any money, and it could give you a huge personal or financial return. Just stop wasting it!

# DEVELOPING YOUR TIME SKILLS

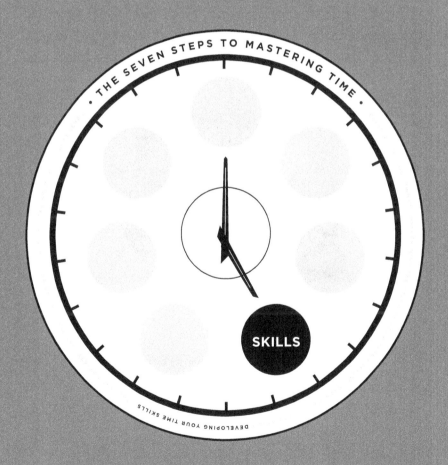

THE SEVEN STEPS TO MASTERING TIME

SKILLS

DEVELOPING YOUR TIME SKILLS

While some people may have the right motivation to become time masters, and others feel the need to change, the process also requires skills.

There are many examples of this in daily life, including sports. Regardless of how much you love the game of baseball, if you want to play well you need to be skillful in hitting, fielding, throwing, catching, and running. These may not require superman talents, but they are skills to master.

Successful time mastery also involves developing skills and ongoing practice.

The first belief is that 80 percent of time success is a science and 20 percent is an art. This is important to believe because you are giving yourself the permission to get better if you choose. You were not born to be a time master.

# SUCCESS =

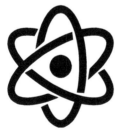 

*80% Science*              *20% Art*

You can have the right beliefs and change what you are doing but you also need time skills to be successful. Planning is a skill.

Another important formula to become more skillful is: A + B = R

For many people, achieving success is an outcome. But those who achieve success realize that the outcome is just a product of doing certain things. The formula to achieve the success outcome is:

# A (attitude) + B (behavior) = R (results)

If you focus on the attitude and the behaviors the results will follow.

For example:

| | | |
|---|---|---|
| A (attitude) | = | the right mind-set |
| A | = | positive attitude |
| A | = | work ethic |
| A | = | discipline |
| B (behavior) | = | getting skills |
| B | = | gaining knowledge |
| B | = | following a process consistently |
| R (results) | = | the goal/outcome |

Developing the right attitude and the right behaviors are just like working on any other skills. You just need to identify them and then work on a plan to improve them.

The following are some key skills for time mastery.

## VISUALIZING TIME: IF YOU CAN SEE IT . . . YOU GET IT

Based on my experience training thousands of individuals in business improvement, sales, and marketing, I would say most people are visual thinkers. They understand better when they can visualize something. If I simply talk about basic concepts or processes, often I am met with glazed stares. If I supplement my talk with an image or a diagram illustrating the same concept, the comprehension and understanding increases significantly. And if they understand it, they can master it.

Visualization can involve very literal images, or it can be about tapping into our experiences through analogies or metaphors. The use of metaphors and analogies can help the person you are trying to communicate with understand more easily. For example, I talk about the four quarters of a football game. If a team is ahead twenty to zero after the first quarter, they are probably not going to abandon their game plan. On the other hand, if the halftime score is zero to twenty, the strategy dramatically changes. For people who understand football, they immediately get this concept of how urgency could affect how you look at time.

There are many visual experiences that relate to understanding time, such as driving speed or the dashboard on a car. It can also be wandering lost in a maze, not knowing where you are going and the inefficiency of that. Time-related analogies can also work with cooking or exercise (e.g., taking something out of the oven too soon).

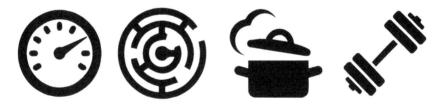

*Visualizations of time-related experiences.*

The more you can visualize time and make translating time visually into a skill, the more you will be able to understand it, leverage it, and manipulate it to be more effective.

There are many other simple visual ways to think about time.

### 1. The traditional clock.

By seeing time as a circle, you can comprehend an hour or a twelve-hour half-day better. There is a beginning and end. There is a cycle to it. Children need to see the numbers on a clock as a way to learn, but as people get older, most can begin to feel the time in quarter or halves or the complete circle. While very simple, it is a good example of making time visual.

## 2. Timeline.

By visualizing time in a linear fashion, you see both the relationship (what needs to come first/middle/last) between activities and the volume of time each activity takes. Timelines are often used in days or weeks, but they can be equally effective on the scale of one day or even one hour. I like to use a "reverse timeline" when helping someone work though the activities and tasks required to achieve a deadline. By making it more visual and tangible, you can actually see how difficult or easy it will be to achieve the goal.

## 3. Calendar.

With the advent of technology and the increased use of online scheduling, many people have gotten away from some basic uses of the printed calendar. A common calendar allows you to see the relationships of the day, week, month, and year. It also helps you measure how urgent certain tasks are and when you have blocks of time to work on things that might be overwhelming you. While I find new technologies helpful I also use a simple traditional day timer so I can better see the weeks and months visually.

## 4. A Gantt chart.

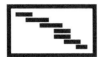 Another less familiar but common time visual-izer is a Gantt chart (invented by Henry Laurence Gantt in the early 1900s). This tool is used to map projects that have interdependent activities. It helps the user see the flow of the project, identifies opportunities to save or reduce time, and highlights critical tasks that need to be accomplished at a certain time. Using methodologies like this in other areas not only helps give you a better result but also helps you further understand time and the relationships between activities.

## 5. A metaphor.

 "If a picture is worth a thousand words, a metaphor is worth a thousand pictures." Most of us communicate daily using metaphors. Some people use them to be clever, but most use them to simply try to communicate ideas and themes. By thinking of metaphors that relate to time, you can visualize time better and therefore understand many of the impacts of time, such as urgency, importance of planning, and short-term versus long-term time. If you are a sports fan, find a time metaphor in football or tennis. If you enjoy cooking, begin to think of a baking or cooking metaphor that relates to time. Any area (like fishing or flying or driving) has potential metaphors that are useful in understanding and communicating time. Try to think of a few. Make a game out of it over dinner with your family and they will become more top of mind. The key to using metaphors is finding a relevant topic that will help you see and understand time better. And again, if you see it you will get it.

As you become more masterful with time-visualization tools, you will elevate your understanding. With greater understanding, time will become more important to you. And when that happens, your mental time muscles will become stronger.

## ESTIMATING TIME

To become more masterful managing your time, you must condition your estimating time "muscle". I refer to it as a muscle more than a skill because, like muscle in your body, the more you use it, the stronger they become.

Being able to estimate time has several elements to it.

1. **A mind-set.** Begin thinking about how much time things take and visually connecting the dots between time and an activity. It will improve your estimating-time skill but also creates more meaning and value in the activity.

2. **Practice.** Like any other muscle, it needs to be active, not static or passive. Practicing time estimation can be painful or uncomfortable for some people. Like other physical exercises, once you do it regularly, it can be fun and fulfilling. You might even get the runner's (time estimator's) high if you work it.

3. **Courage.** When I ask people to estimate the time it takes for a task, one of the biggest obstacles is the fear of being wrong. When you are fearful of something you tend to be paralyzed and not do or think about it. I often then ask, "What is the worst thing about being wrong?" It's not really a big deal. So get out of your comfort zone and guess more, then see how close you are (it might even become fun). This courage will lead to being better and more skillful.

When I began my career in the remodeling business, I had to estimate the time many things would take. How long would it take to build a wall or tear out a bathroom? How much time would be required to design and develop a plan for an addition to a home? How many meetings would be required to make all the design decisions and come to closure on a construction contract? Estimating these activities not only made me more knowledgeable at estimating time; it also helped me develop the estimating-time muscles to apply it to other daily activities. Once you begin to really see the benefits of this subject, you practice it more, and you begin to have fun with it too.

The following are a few tips that will allow you to begin to sharpen your estimating skills and improve in this important time-mastery topic.

1. **Guess and then measure it.** Begin with some simple tasks like making breakfast in the morning, getting ready for work, or doing your exercise routine. While it may sound a little mechanical, write down the number of minutes you think it takes to do some routine tasks. Then check the amount of time it actually takes. For example, it takes me five minutes to make breakfast, and it takes me twelve minutes to do my morning routine. By beginning to do these simple time exercises, you will improve your estimating skills/muscles. After thinking about the simple daily tasks, expand your estimating: How long will it take for an effective meeting or for a project to be completed? Don't be paralyzed by fear of being wrong. If you guess, that will lead to being more knowledgeable, which will in turn lead to the confidence needed to estimate time. This is an important skill if you are going to master time.

2. **Question the amount of time it takes.** Ask yourself, "Are there ways to save time in this process?" Just by asking the question, you will not only be more conscious of the time but also should be able to find ways to improve and save some time. I was able to save ninety seconds in making my coffee, which is about ten hours per year. Don't get too obsessed by the questioning; but by asking, your knowledge and sensitivity in estimating time will increase.

3. **Make it a game.** I often will do time games with people when discussing subjects like this. Ask a family member or friend to estimate time for any familiar task. For example, "How much time does it take to watch a baseball game on TV without the commercials?" or "How much time does it take to shop at the grocery store?" This may not be a game where there is a winner or loser, but it does allow you to see how time-sensitive that person is or how good they are at estimating time.

4. **List things that take about the same amount of time.** Another exercise that helps improve your estimating muscles is to list a few amounts of time and then list three activities that roughly can fit that amount of time; for example: ten minutes = a short dog walk / a shower / calling my sister; thirty minutes = going and getting my hair cut / a longer dog walk / making dinner; sixty minutes = driving to work / a lunch with a business friend / a healthy workout; four hours = a drive to the beach / building a set of shelves / a movie and dinner. By beginning to estimate the time things take and then comparing them to others things, you not only improve the estimating skills but you also begin

to think about time in terms of equivalent activities. Do this with activities that are important to *you*.

5. **Make estimating time more visual.** As discussed earlier, I believe most people are visual thinkers. If you can begin to see the time visually, you can also estimate it better. For example, draw a line on a piece of paper. This line represents eight hours. Now make a circle at the beginning and then the end of the line and a circle in the middle so you now have two parts representing four-hour segments. Then add a circle just a short distance from one end. This now represents an hour. Now begin to see your day in this line. Begin to estimate activities that fit into the time slots.

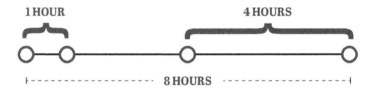

Another way to estimate time visually is by using a pie chart, as discussed in the earlier chapter. The pie chart represents a day and can be used to estimate (and illustrate) the five to seven categories of activities (personal and professional) that will make up the day. Is this an ideal amount of time? Are there ways you can improve it or reallocate some time for other things? In a later chapter, I talk about a "stress-cloud" exercise later to help visualize and reduce stress. If you think about time as a cloud (estimating big chunks of time as big clouds that don't let the sun come in and small ones as just passing or scattered clouds), you begin to see not only why you are feeling the way you are (in a funk) and also ways to break up the cloud and let the sun come in. There are many ways to estimate time visually, but you just need to begin with drawing a line.

Not being able to accurately estimate time is like approaching the subject of time mastery in the dark or flying blind or trying to run a race with a broken leg. If you can become more conscious of how long things can take, you are on a good path towards becoming more masterful.

Three things to close with:

1. **Estimate it**

2. **See it**

3. **Control it**

Then you will begin to master time.

## ANALYZING TIME

Another skill or muscle that you need to use and improve upon is analysis. This begins with asking the right questions. I generally encourage people to ask themselves these five questions to begin the process:

1. *Why am I doing this?*

2. *Is there a better way to do it?*

3. *Am I moving my longer-term goals forward?*

4. *Is there a way to delegate this effectively?*

5. *Is this an aggressive but realistic pace?*

After meaningful questions, try to use some visualization techniques and tools to see the answer.

For example, I did a deep analysis of the amount of time I spent traveling in 2016. I made, on average, three trips every two weeks. Some were short and some were longer. I then figured the amount of unproductive time relating to travel (cabs, security lines, an occasional delayed flight, boarding process, paperwork, travel arrangements, etc.) I determined that an average trip had seven hours of time that was unproductive (as well as stressful or boring). I then multiplied that by the number of trips (about seventy-five) in the year. This gave me 525 unproductive hours in the year. So I determined if I could reduce the number of trips to forty, I would save 245 unproductive hours. To express this in equivalent terms, in 245 hours I was able to write this book, develop a podcast series, and walk my dog three times a week.

Without this simple analysis, I would not have appreciated the wasted time and how I could invest it more positively.

This is a process. It's a skill that you need to develop if you want to be more time-masterful.

**The analysis process:**

1. **Take inventory of the numbers** (hours/ROI/blends).

2. **Ask the right questions** (write it down).

3. **Determine a solution** (diagram and make a plan).

The more you can make the analysis visual, the better you will see the road map to success. Once you have done this, you realize that by just investing the time to study the data you will glean important solutions and better answers.

# TIME MYTHS

**I need to set an alarm clock.** Most people use an alarm clock—but I have not used one since 1992. When you become more acute at estimating time, you can just tell yourself when you need to wake up, and your body will do it for you. I am not sure how this works, but I do believe there are time muscles that we need to use. We especially see this in animals, like our pets. My dog Charlie wakes up at precisely the same time every day. He knows exactly when it is time (6:00 p.m.) for his dinner. Again, I am not a doctor or a scientist, but if you begin to consciously think about time, your ability to be aware of it and control it improves.

## MAKING APPOINTMENTS WITH YOURSELF

While this is a simple act, it is also a skill and a habit. You may have heard the biblical commandment, "Thou shalt love thy neighbor as thyself." Some people read this and think it is about being nice and kind to others. However, it can also be interpreted as saying that loving yourself is important, too. While you might think of this as a mind-set more than a skill, I think the most successful people believe they are important—and you need to treat yourself with the same degree of reverence as you do others.

I make this part of the time-mastery process skills because, when we boil it all down, it is about making time for *you*. I include it in the planning process because if you don't make these appointments with yourself, improvement does not happen. We've been told it is strange to talk to ourselves—but talking to myself is critical to success. And I must admit I love making appointments with myself.

| | SUN | MON | TUE | WED | THU | FRI | SAT |
|---|---|---|---|---|---|---|---|
| 8 am | | Plan next mo. sales targets | | | | | |
| 9 am | | | | | | Work on computer skills | |
| 10 am | | | | | | | |
| 11 am | | | | | | | |
| 12 pm | | | | | Lunch with advisor | | |
| 1 pm | | | | | | | |
| 2 pm | | | | | | | |
| 3 pm | | | | | | | |
| 4 pm | | | | Develop top 10 ideas for summer | | | |
| 5 pm | | | | | | | |
| 6 pm | | | | | | | |

You can make appointments (and block it out in your week and day) to do regular things like exercise or walk the dog. You can also make appointments (even small ones, twenty to thirty minutes) with yourself to focus on various ways you want to improve. I often create a meeting with myself to think about a topic or issue that needs attention, such as an issue with a family member or a team-member question to contemplate.

On a very practical basis I find it is best to highlight in advance a few of these mini-appointments. Then on the day-of brain dump, include this as an item: "Mark: top fun things for this summer." Then estimate the amount of time you want to think or work on this (say twenty minutes) and build it into the day's design just like you would any other item.

Because this is a meeting with yourself you should treat it as important as any other meeting—without interruptions, at a designated time, and with the thoughts documented.

Again some may say this is a mind-set more than a skill, but if you develop the techniques and fine-tune them, it is hugely valuable to feeling better and more fulfilled.

# THE TIME-MASTERY SYSTEM

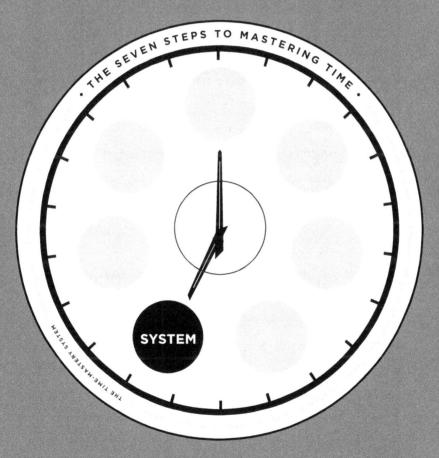

*The future starts today, not tomorrow.*

POPE JOHN PAUL II

In earlier chapters, I established the importance of time management. I have also given you new ways to think about time. Some of you have already begun to take serious inventory of how you are spending your time and where the opportunities for improvement lie. This system pulls together everything you have read so far. If you need to go back and skim the themes and chapters, it might help bring the following time-mastery system to life.

Now this is where the secret sauce is. I will give you a system to overlay these new thoughts and insights into an actual daily plan or tool. The plan is a blueprint, like an architectural design, which, when followed correctly, will allow you to accomplish more, keep promises, and be less overwhelmed and stressed. The goal is to be in control of your day rather than letting your day control you.

I refer to this as a time-mastery system because it is a step-by-step process. The process has a specific order to the steps and it *must* be followed in that order (in the same way that you don't preheat the oven before you buy the ingredients). If you follow these steps properly, you will get results. (Again . . . don't skip steps!) A pilot goes through a specific checklist of steps before taking off, and this results in a 99.99 percent success rate. It is also important to allocate the right amount of time for each step. If you try to do this process too fast, you will not get your desired outcome. There are important dogmatic things, like doing the planning process in the morning, not the night before, and finding a quiet place so you can concentrate fully. These techniques and lessons have come from many years of experimenting and coaching people who have adopted this successfully.

I also created a workbook that you can use for the first thirty days. The workbook is like having training wheels while learning to ride a bike. Once the system becomes part of your daily routine, you can use your own spiral notebook. Again, this is a little dogmatic, but it needs to be a spiral notebook. And you need to handwrite rather than use your computer.

There are several parts to the system, and I will walk you through them. First, read through the entire system to get an overview, then go back and use the book like a recipe to follow. There are other tools like the time-mastery system audio and video tools that can help you understand things better, connect the dots, and fine-tune your techniques.

# THE TIME-MASTERY SYSTEM OUTLINE

| 1 | THE SETUP |
|---|---|
| 2 | THE BRAIN DUMP |
| 3 | ESTIMATING THE TIME |
| 4 | TIMELINE SETUP |
| 5 | CONNECTING THE ACTIVITIES TO THE TIMELINE |
| 6 | ANALYZING THE PRELIMINARY PLAN |
| 7 | FINAL PLAN |
| 8 | LAUNCH |
| 9 | MONITORING THE JOURNEY |
| 10 | ADJUSTING THE PLAN |

## THE SETUP

The setup is the preparation step. This involves physical, environmental, and mental preparation. If you start the time-mastery system without the right environment, you will fail. If you don't have all your information for your day at your fingertips, you will create a weak plan. If you are distracted and not mentally focused when you begin, you will find the process painful and ineffective. Here are some basic keys for the setup step.

1. **Find a quiet place to do the time-mastery system (TMS).** It needs to be at the *beginning* of your day. If you do this process the night before, the design will be flawed. Things happen mysteriously overnight to change what your day's plan should be. The setting to plan could be in your home,

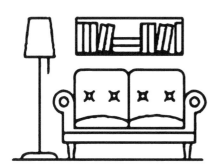

your office, or even in a park or quiet corner of a coffee shop. If you do it in your home, it should not be at the breakfast table with your family. If it is in your office, you may need to find a quiet conference room to get away from the normal early-morning distractions at your desk. A friend who I once coached simply moved his setup location away from his office and became more successful with the system. If you're a person who works better at night, I recommend you create a to-do list at night and review it again in the morning.

2. **Have all your planning information at your fingertips.** This includes your calendar, saved voicemails, e-mails, text messages, and any other notes that might be useful. Think

of these as the ingredients you will assemble for a meal. If you are missing some, you will have a flawed outcome.

3.  **Have enough time to plan.** I generally advise people to do the TMS at least sixty minutes before their first scheduled activity or meeting. For example, if you have a conference call at 8:30 a.m., make sure you are sitting down doing the TMS at or before 7:30 a.m. If your first meeting is at 10 a.m., you have some flexibility, but doing it at 7:30 a.m. is fine too. A rushed design is a flawed design.

# TIME MYTHS

**I don't have time to plan.** This is one of the more common and painful misconceptions. I would say you don't have time *not* to plan. Planning is the key to finding large bonus dividends of time. Unfortunately, planning does take a little time. Some people try to do a daily plan in fifteen or twenty minutes and fail. You need a minimum of thirty minutes a day to plan. It is sort of like cooking time. Some things take thirty minutes to bake in the oven. If you take them out too early, they are not done and taste bad. If you leave things in too long, they will burn and also taste bad. By investing the minimum of thirty minutes, you will—after a week or two of using this system—realize a dividend of one to two hours of found time a day.

4. **Use the TMS notebook (or a spiral notebook).** While this may sound a little old fashioned, it is *critical* to your success. Most of the time when I follow up with students of the system who are struggling, I find it is simple things like not using a spiral notebook that is derailing them. This notebook will be the blueprint that you carry with you throughout the day. It becomes a tool to document your thoughts so you can think more clearly and efficiently. Your TMS plan needs to be monitored frequently, and you need to have your notebook with you to do that.

5. **The first week or two will be awkward (and a little tough).** As I teach and present this system, most participants say it makes complete sense and they want to adopt it. Even people who struggle with the system initially will—after the first week—begin to see benefits like reduced stress and increased accomplishments. As with any lifestyle adjustment (like that first tough week of running), it takes time to instill new behavior. Try to be patient with the system and yourself.

# THE TEMPLATE

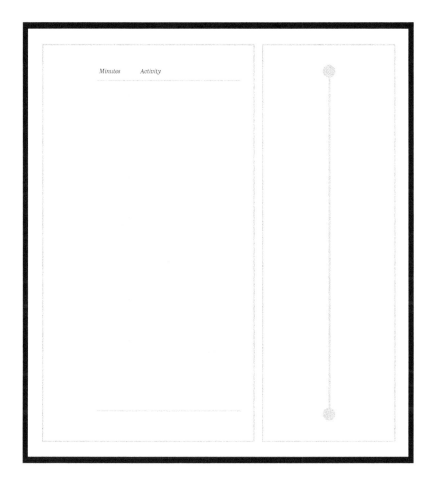

*Minutes*   *Activity*

*Success or failure is often determined
on the drawing board.*

R OBERT M CKAIN

## BRAIN DUMP

The brain dump is a deeper version of most people's "to-do" list.

To begin this process, I generally like to have a "theme" for the day. It can be philosophical like "be happy" or tactical like "close the deal." While some people find this less important, I find that having some directional theme for the day helps as you work through the planning process—and is helpful to keep you on track throughout the day.

Next, begin to do your brain dump (a deep to-do list). Write down as many personal and professional things as fast as you can that you need to do that day (and *only* that day). Your brain flows much faster than your hand can write, so try to abbreviate as you dump. Expand on each item as required with a couple of additional bullets that will help you understand the scope of what needs to be done, to help you better estimate the time later. If an item is a phone call, you might highlight a couple of things you want to discuss on that call. Have your calendar and other tools at your fingertips so that your brain dump can be very comprehensive. I am often asked, "How do you know when you are done with the brain dump?" It is simple. You are done when there is nothing left to dump out of your brain *for that day*. It is important to only list the items for that day. (If other thoughts pop up, just put them on a separate paper to add to your calendar for another day.) Over time this will become an easier and more natural process.

After you have somewhere between twelve and twenty-two items for your daily brain dump, take a brief "time out." Stand up; get a

| Minutes | Activity |
|---------|----------|
| | Lunch |
| | Set... BM/JH/JA/MK |
| | Call John - SL Training |
| | JS mtg. sales profile system |
| | Meeting with Smith |
| | MK Card |
| | BM one on one |
| | Call GM; lease, trip, agenda |
| | Miller contract review |
| | ME B-Day |
| | Call Jim |
| | Set PM (Kit. Mtg.) |
| | Call Tom K (Oregon) |
| | CK w/WJFK schedule |
| | Call TB sales/vm/temp |
| | Reactive Time (Misc.) |
| | New Training Concept |
| | Set JR Lunch |

*Fig. 1 — Brain Dump*

cup of coffee or a glass of water. Walk outside for a minute and get some fresh air. While you are doing this, ask yourself:

- *"Is there anything else I would like to accomplish today?"*

- *"Is there something in my longer-term plan I can inch forward today?"*

- *"Is there anyone else I can contact or help today?"*

By asking yourself these three questions, you will likely come up with a few additional items to add to your brain dump. Now you should have around fourteen to twenty-five items on your brain-dump list. If you have fewer than that, you might want to go a little deeper. If you have more, you might want to move some to another day or look for ways to combine/leverage them. At this point in the process, most people feel this is not hugely dissimilar from the to-do list process they currently do (just a little more structured).

Now add one very important item labeled "reactive time" to your brain dump list. I will explain this concept more.

Now the real planning starts.

## ESTIMATING THE TIME

The next step in the process is to estimate the amount of minutes each task or activity will take. This process should be written on the left side of the brain dump items (see example). This is an estimation. Over time you will get better and more skillful at predicting time.

Use five minutes as the smallest increment of time, even for tasks that will only take a minute or two to complete. Try to be realistic with your estimates (not too conservative or liberal). If you are struggling or it is difficult to estimate, just guess—then use this as a placeholder to review a little later. The estimating-time step should only take five minutes. It may not be the same stream of consciousness as the brain dump, but don't labor over it. Just do a quick educated guess.

For example:

- *10 min. . . . call JR*

- *5 min. . . . set meeting with josh*

- *60 min. . . . meeting with SM . . . trip / DB / 2018 thoughts*

"Reactive time" is not something you can estimate. During the first thirty days, allow for 120 minutes of reactive time. This time is very important to plan for, but you cannot predict when it will happen.

Now add up all the minutes and write the sum down at the bottom. Then divide by sixty to give the number of hours needed to complete all the activities. Then compare that number to the overall hours available in that day. For instance, if it adds up to 9.75 hours and that day is 8:00 a.m. to 6:00 p.m. that equals ten hours—so it works! If, however, it adds up to twelve hours and you have ten hours

| Minutes | Activity |
|---|---|
| 20 | Lunch |
| 20 | Set... BM/JH/JA/MK |
| 30 | Call John - SL Training |
| 60 | JS mtg. sales profile system |
| 90 | Meeting with Smith |
| 15 | MK Card |
| 60 | BM one on one |
| 30 | Call GM; lease, trip, agenda |
| 30 | Miller contract review |
| 10 | ME B-Day |
| 5 | Call Jim |
| 20 | Set PM (Kit. Mtg.) |
| 35 | Call Tom K (Oregon) |
| 30 | CK w/WJFK schedule |
| 60 | Call TB sales/vm/temp |
| 120 | Reactive Time (Misc.) |
| 30 | New Training Concept |
| 10 | Set JR Lunch |

675 min / 60 = **11.25 hrs.**

Fig. 2 — Estimating the Time

available, then it does not work, and you need to go back and massage the brain dump and estimated time.

Ask yourself if there is another way to do the activity. Can you do an outline today and then finish the proposal tomorrow when it is due? There will be many days in the beginning that these numbers do not align closely. (For example, if you have 14.5 hours of activities for an eleven-hour day.) If this is the case, see instructions for common mistakes, which are listed later in this chapter. But never move forward without first getting the estimated time to align with the time available in the day.

## TIMELINE SETUP

Since most of us are visual thinkers, the timeline helps make your day more visual. This timeline is linear as shown in the example on the following page. When setting this up, follow these simple steps:

1.  **Draw a line as noted (or use the TMS notebook template).**

2.  **Have a beginning and an end. This represents your day. (Launch at 8:00 a.m. and finish at 5:30 p.m.) Draw a circle at these end points.**

3.  **Create the other points based on that specific day's activities (e.g., a 10:00 a.m. to 11:00 a.m. meeting; lunch at noon to 12:30 p.m.).**

4.  **Try to keep intervals no more than three hours. If you have a larger gap, try to break it up into two or three parts.**

5.  **Now reflect on this diagram. Can you begin to see and feel the structure that makes sense in your day?**

6.  **Make the minor adjustments for the right balance. Each day will vary between five to ten blocks of time, which is why each day is unique and needs to be customized rather than using a standard template.**

7. Now, block out (or color in) the blocks of times where you have a meeting, conference call, or appointment— again to visualize the day.

8. Now create a letter (symbol) for each time section (A, B, C, etc.).

9. The draft of the timeline is complete.

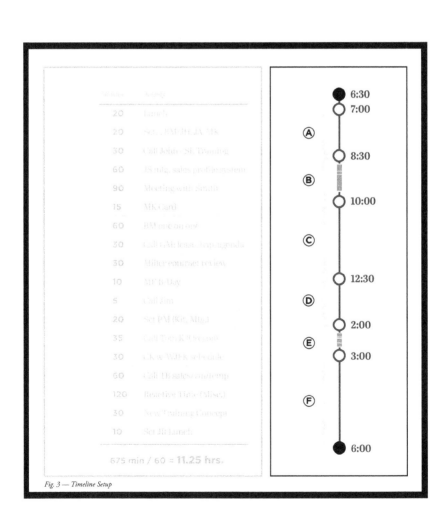

*Fig. 3 — Timeline Setup*

## CONNECT THE BRAIN-DUMP ITEMS TO THE TIMELINE

Now connect the dots between the timeline and the activities list. This step requires thought. Begin with the obvious ones, such as meetings or conference calls. Then think about when in the day you will be in the best frame of mind or have the right urgency to get individual items done. You will have some filler items that can be done anytime—but you need to fit them into the time slot available. This step may sound very simple, but don't rush it. Slow down and think of ways to leverage and multitask to gain valuable minutes.

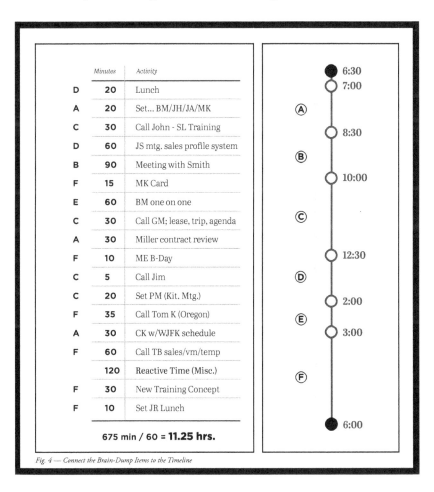

Fig. 4 — Connect the Brain-Dump Items to the Timeline

## ANALYSIS

Now let's take time to do a simple analysis. Add up all the individual time sections and write them on the left side of the timeline. Then see if they fit the time allowed (e.g., the A = eighty minutes, which fits in a ninety-minute time slot). If they don't (which is common), just move an activity to another time slot or modify the activity's goal so it will fit. Keep in mind that there is some reactive time that will unavoidably slip into time slots, so it is always best to have some wiggle room. *Do not move forward unless everything fits and works.*

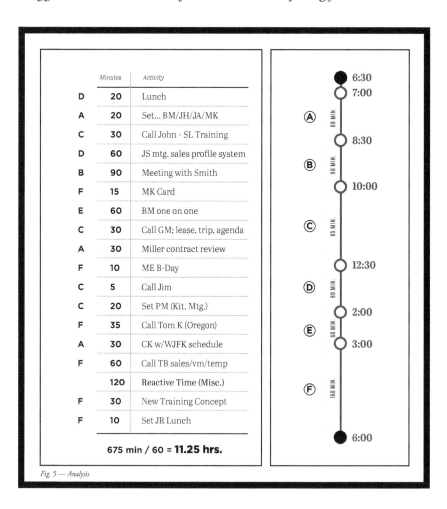

|   | Minutes | Activity |
|---|---------|----------|
| D | 20 | Lunch |
| A | 20 | Set... BM/JH/JA/MK |
| C | 30 | Call John - SL Training |
| D | 60 | JS mtg. sales profile system |
| B | 90 | Meeting with Smith |
| F | 15 | MK Card |
| E | 60 | BM one on one |
| C | 30 | Call GM; lease, trip, agenda |
| A | 30 | Miller contract review |
| F | 10 | ME B-Day |
| C | 5 | Call Jim |
| C | 20 | Set PM (Kit. Mtg.) |
| F | 35 | Call Tom K (Oregon) |
| A | 30 | CK w/WJFK schedule |
| F | 60 | Call TB sales/vm/temp |
|   | 120 | Reactive Time (Misc.) |
| F | 30 | New Training Concept |
| F | 10 | Set JR Lunch |

675 min / 60 = **11.25 hrs.**

Timeline:
- 6:30
- 7:00
- (A) 80 MIN.
- 8:30
- (B) 90 MIN.
- 10:00
- (C) 85 MIN.
- 12:30
- (D) 80 MIN.
- 2:00
- (E) 60 MIN.
- 3:00
- (F) 160 MIN.
- 6:00

*Fig. 5 — Analysis*

Here are a few important questions to ask yourself before the launch.

The blueprint or road map for your day:

a. Does it work (i.e., do the times fit the activities)?

b. Is this plan aggressive but realistic?

c. Are the activities/pace consistent with your theme and goals for the day?

## THE LAUNCH

Congratulations! You now have a blueprint for your day. Take a minute and review it. Try to think about what is missing. Ask yourself, "Is it too aggressive or too conservative?" Before long, you will find the right cadence for you.

Now focus on *only* the A items. Pick any A you want to focus on. And do it! Circle each item as you complete it and then move on to the next one. Think about "aggressive-but-realistic" pace. If you complete all the As and have extra time, grab an item from another time slot and just get it done, or use the little gaps of time to deal with reactive things that pop up. You never know exactly when you might slip with some reactive activities later in the day.

## MONITORING YOUR PLAN

The most common mistake made with this and other systems is not *monitoring* your plan throughout the day. You will need to monitor it every sixty to ninety minutes. It is easy to make minor adjustments if you  know early where you are off or ahead of your plan. This monitoring process will get easier over time. If you get used to carrying the notebook with you, you can do the monitoring in the little gaps of time throughout the day. Use the little gaps of time to monitor.

## ADJUSTING YOUR PLAN

While we all hope the day will give you what you planned, unfortunately, it probably will not. You need to build in a process to adjust your game plan. It helps again here to think about football. A good coach does not throw out his game plan after the first ten minutes

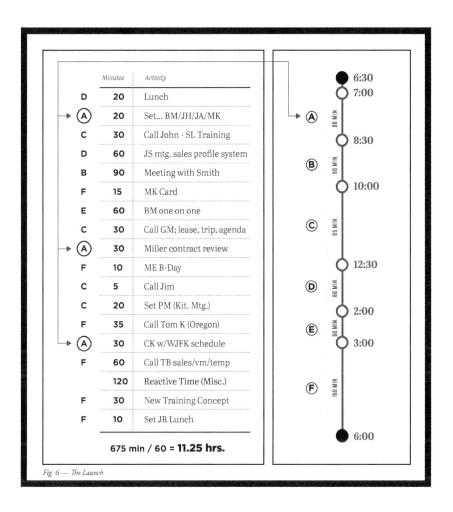

| | Minutes | Activity |
|---|---|---|
| D | 20 | Lunch |
| (A) | 20 | Set... BM/JH/JA/MK |
| C | 30 | Call John - SL Training |
| D | 60 | JS mtg. sales profile system |
| B | 90 | Meeting with Smith |
| F | 15 | MK Card |
| E | 60 | BM one on one |
| C | 30 | Call GM; lease, trip, agenda |
| (A) | 30 | Miller contract review |
| F | 10 | ME B-Day |
| C | 5 | Call Jim |
| C | 20 | Set PM (Kit. Mtg.) |
| F | 35 | Call Tom K (Oregon) |
| (A) | 30 | CK w/WJFK schedule |
| F | 60 | Call TB sales/vm/temp |
| | 120 | Reactive Time (Misc.) |
| F | 30 | New Training Concept |
| F | 10 | Set JR Lunch |

**675 min / 60 = 11.25 hrs.**

Timeline:
- 6:30
- 7:00
- (A) 80 MIN
- 8:30
- (B) 90 MIN
- 10:00
- (C) 85 MIN
- 12:30
- (D) 80 MIN
- 2:00
- (E) 60 MIN
- 3:00
- (F) 160 MIN
- 6:00

*Fig. 6 — The Launch*

into the game when he is down by three points. However, at halftime he'll take a serious (and quick) inventory of what's working or not, what the score is, and what the team needs to do in the second half.

Adjusting your time game plan or design is very similar. As you monitor every sixty to ninety minutes, you are making minor tweaks and adjustments. Then, at midday, I encourage you to make a real halftime adjustment. (I generally can do this in a few minutes, so you don't need to make it an event, but in the first thirty days, allow ten minutes for halftime planning.) This halftime adjustment looks at what has been accomplished. It looks at any changes in the goals for the day. It also addresses the things that have popped up and might need to be planned for directly or scheduled for another day.

Again, this planning system is dynamic and a tool that you adjust and manipulate as you go.

I always take a few minutes at the end of each day and review what I accomplished. I look at what requires planning notes or scheduling for future days—and then generally I smile and take a deep breath after having a very successful and productive day.

# COMMON MISTAKES PEOPLE MAKE

*Lost time is never found again.*

BENJAMIN FRANKLIN

Most students of success understand that it can be achieved by being skillful or clever—but also simply by eliminating or avoiding mistakes. For example, when taking a trip, your goal may be to get to your destination safely. If you are driving, you need to avoid accidents and car trouble to arrive safely. So how do you achieve this? You drive defensively by leaving adequate space between cars, you take your car in for regular maintenance, and you avoid potholes or debris in the road. This is a simplistic example, but it also holds true when mastering the TMS. Avoid potential potholes and the likelihood of success increases.

The following are the seven most-common mistakes people make with this TMS.

## 1. Forcing fourteen hours into a ten-hour day

This is like pouring a quart of milk into a pint jar. It does not work. So why do we attempt this when it comes to our day? Since you are estimating the amount of time things will take, you might be overly optimistic about how long something will take. It might also be you are overwhelmed and believe if everything miraculously got done, life would be wonderful. Or it could be that you are not allowing or anticipating enough inevitable reactive time in your day. The bottom line is that ninety-five times out of a hundred, you are setting yourself up for failure. It is critical that the time estimated to do your activities is closely aligned with the time allowed for the day, and fourteen hours is

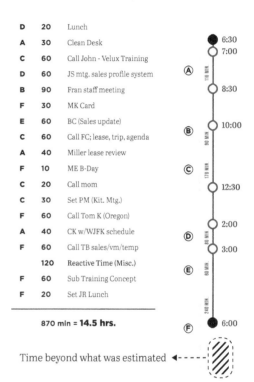

| | | |
|---|---|---|
| D | 20 | Lunch |
| A | 30 | Clean Desk |
| C | 60 | Call John - Velux Training |
| D | 60 | JS mtg. sales profile system |
| B | 90 | Fran staff meeting |
| F | 30 | MK Card |
| E | 60 | BC (Sales update) |
| C | 60 | Call FC; lease, trip, agenda |
| A | 40 | Miller lease review |
| F | 10 | ME B-Day |
| C | 20 | Call mom |
| C | 30 | Set PM (Kit. Mtg.) |
| F | 60 | Call Tom K (Oregon) |
| A | 40 | CK w/WJFK schedule |
| F | 60 | Call TB sales/vm/temp |
| | 120 | Reactive Time (Misc.) |
| F | 60 | Sub Training Concept |
| F | 20 | Set JR Lunch |

870 min = **14.5 hrs.**

Time beyond what was estimated

not even close! As illustrated here, you need to go back and work your brain-dump activities. Ask if there are other ways to communicate or accomplish the task in a shorter amount of time. I prefer not to push things completely to the next day. You may want to break an item down so you can at least inch it forward today, then complete it on a future day.

## 2. Doing your TMS planning in the wrong place/time

Here's a simple checklist to successful planning. If the answer to any of these is no, then fix it, or you will likely fail.

a. **Is it quiet enough for you to concentrate?** (Not at the breakfast table with the kids or in a place you get interrupted, like a crowded office.)

b. **Do you have enough time (a minimum of thirty minutes) to properly plan?** If you only have fifteen minutes, it is a rough sketch of your day—not a plan.

c. **Is it in the morning—not the evening before?** (Some things happen overnight that can make your design flawed.)

## 3. Not monitoring

This is a journey that requires a map to help you navigate successfully. By reviewing your design every sixty to ninety minutes, you are making sure you don't miss an exit. If you have a detour in your journey (and you will), you can make minor adjustments to reach your destination or goal. Always carry your notebook with you so you can use the little gaps of time to monitor your progress.

## 4. Allowing for too many interruptions

While you don't want to be rude or disrespectful, it is essential that you treat yourself with the same level of importance and reverence that you treat others. When someone interrupts you, consider asking if you can address his or her issue on your schedule rather than immediately dropping everything. This is a well-planned journey, and if you are constantly interrupted, you will never reach your destination on time. Go back to the reactive versus proactive chapter and try to improve with the techniques.

## 5. Brain-dump items are too general

There is an important balance for your brain-dump items. You don't want them to be too detailed (e.g., "fill my coffee cup"), but the more common mistake is making them too broad. Consider breaking a larger item into several smaller parts. For example, listing "Work on the Jones project" would be too broad to accurately estimate the time required. A better approach is to break the larger item into several smaller tasks:

    a.   Jones outline *(twenty minutes)*

    b.   Jones rough draft *(forty minutes)*

    c.   Get feedback on draft from Mary *(twenty minutes)*

By breaking an item into parts, you will be able to better estimate the time required. You also may be able to accomplish some parts at different times of the day rather than in one sitting.

## 6. Getting too creative

I am a creative person, but you don't need to be to make the TMS work for you. A common mistake is that creative people want to modify or tweak my system. They like to cross things out rather than circle the letters. They try to be efficient by developing a template for the design that can save them time. They do the techniques at night versus in the morning. I can go on and on, but the message is this: for the first thirty days follow these techniques. 100 percent! When people struggle or fall off the wagon, it is generally because they veer off the road by getting too creative.

### 7. Giving up too soon

The first week is tough for everyone. You are changing your basic daily patterns. You are using muscles that you may not be used to using. Before beginning this process, you still filled your day with something that took thirty or forty minutes, and now you are adding to an already busy schedule. The reason I ask for a thirty-day commitment is that, like any other habit, it takes twenty to thirty days to establish the behavior. I also know you will feel much better and begin to accomplish the "why" goals. Once you experience some control over your day and see the ROI, you will continue to be vested into the system. Don't give up too soon!

This system does not require an advanced degree or a high level of skill or intelligence. It does require the right mind-set, a little time, and the diligence to stick to it.

---

# THE TOP-TEN TMS QUESTIONS ANSWERED

### 1. Do I need to do this planning process over the weekend?

No. I find most people have a very different rhythm or cadence over the weekend. Some like to surrender control to their family or their personal life, or just go with the flow and let the day control them. Others just need to recharge. For those who need a more structured plan over the weekend, this planning process (or a slight variation of it) still works. Again, this is a personal planning tool to help you feel better and more fulfilled, not a process to be obsessed with.

## 2. Can I use another type of notebook (a smaller or a fancy binder)?

No. The 8.5" x 11" size is important. You need to be able to see the entire day to massage and work it. You need space to feel like you have room to add notes (which you can refer to the next day). By using a spiral notebook, you will not lose pages, and you can easily refer to a phone number or a note to yourself several days or weeks later. The scale and type of the notebook does matter.

## 3. Can I do this planning process the night before when I have an early meeting the next day?

No, sorry. I recommend getting up thirty minutes earlier to do the process, or wait until after that early meeting to design the rest of the day. I have had many people try doing it the night before, and the results have not been good. Just like when traveling, the weather changes and flights get delayed. You need to do this process in real time. If you have a lot whirling in your head the night before, then just make a mini to-do list that you can use in your planning process the next morning.

### 4. Should I prioritize my brain dump?

Not really. I am a big believer that your brain dump needs to be a "stream-of-consciousness" process. Let the day flow out. Jot down the items as fast as they flow out of your head. After you have everything out and have reviewed your calendar, other tools, notes, etc., then you can manipulate the items and activities to determine whether you want to accomplish them today or not. You also can ask yourself, "When is the best time to accomplish the activities?" I find some of the pressing priorities are like black clouds above you, so you might want to address them early to get the sun to shine in the afternoon.

### 5. What if I am not sure when I should do an item?

This is not a problem. You can always pick two time slots for an item (i.e., B and E). You still need to estimate the time involved the same way. Then you can do it in the time slot that works best in the moment. If you have a list of several minor things, you can also use X, which is time-slot neutral, and then knock these minor items off when you have a few minutes between things.

### 6. What if my brain-dump activities only add up to six hours of time in a ten-hour day?

Although this is rare for me (and most busy people), I generally begin to focus on and stretch my medium- and longer-term muscles. I ask myself if I can move something forward from a future day. I look at my long-term goals and try to inch something forward. I also try to weave more personal interests in when they occur (like a lunch with my daughter or calls to some old friends). Again, it is important to create a plan that fills the day properly (including reactive time), and then work the plan. That is where the fulfillment comes. So find those additional items to fill the day. You will feel better and more fulfilled.

**7. Can I make changes in the plan during the day?**

Yes. You must. You might have an appointment that moves or someone shows up late. You also might need to get in touch with someone you thought you could reach in the morning but were not able to. As discussed, the monitoring and tweaking of the plan is as important as the plan itself. You might make three to seven minor changes and maybe even one or two major changes in the design during the day. Again, this is like a football game. If the score is where you want it to be after the first quarter, then stick to the original plan. If the score is off by a lot, then you adjust your plan. If at halftime, you are down twenty to zero, you need a new game plan for the second half. The dynamic is the same with your day. Monitor and then decide to stick to the plan or adjust it as needed.

**8. How do I weave in a plan for reading and responding to the copious amount of e-mails I get daily?**

The number of e-mails you get can vary quite a bit. I find when I travel, I get 50 percent of the e-mails that I do when I am in my office. I also find that certain days of the week I get more than others. I have surveyed many professional people, and the number of e-mails they receive daily varies from thirty-five to three hundred. The reason I set this in context is that I believe you need to take better control over your e-mails. For example, I did an experiment for a week. As a proactive, friendly guy, I tended to respond to e-mails even when I was not asked to. I decided to try not responding unless asked—and my e-mails dropped by 40 percent. Interesting! Now I have found a balance. Another technique I use is to draft an e-mail then save it and respond later that day in a more thoughtful or careful way (we all know that e-mail responses can be tricky). To go back to the question, if I have several important e-mails to respond to, I would carve out a time (even if only fifteen minutes) to do it. Otherwise, most people can fit them into the reactive time slots available.

### 9. How close does the time for my brain-dump list need to be to the total amount of time available for the day?

My general rule is to not begin the day if there is a thirty-minute or more variance. If you have eleven and a half hours of activities in your brain dump and only ten hours available in your day, then you need to work it more. First go back and make sure you were not too liberal with your time. Then ask if there are better or more effective ways to do some items. Consider shortening a meeting from sixty to fifty minutes. Break a project into parts and move one part into another day (e.g., do a draft today, then the final tomorrow). Is there a different way to accomplish some of the items on your list? Send an e-mail to someone instead of making a more time-consuming phone call. While tweaking will take some time, you want to set yourself up to succeed. So, yes, the plan needs to come very close to the amount of time available in your day.

## 10. What if my day crashes and burns?

Hopefully this will only happen occasionally. It usually is a product of a major fire or just letting it get out of control. The real question is, "How did you feel at the end of the day?" Not great, right? So by being more disciplined and by monitoring more carefully, you will increase the odds of a great day. Before they begin to utilize this system, most people only have one or two good days per week. After using this system, you will increase that to three or four great days per week. If the nature of your work is more firefighting or reactionary, you will have a tough time staying on track. It's important to remember, this is all about improvement, not perfection. So, when this happens, just make sure the next day does not blow up on you too.

# TIME MASTERY IN ACTION

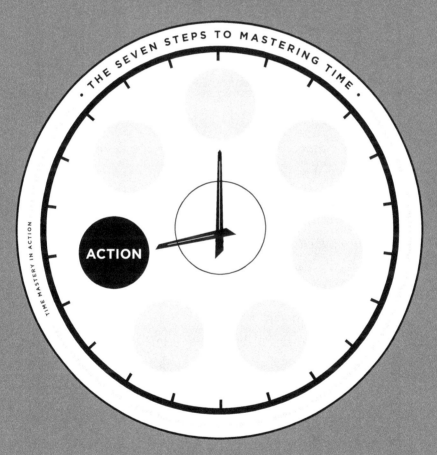

*You can't stop time. You can't capture light. You can only turn your face up and let it rain down.*

KIM EDWARDS

Mastering anything you put your mind to can be the difference between being good and being great. Years ago, I read about the four stages to mastery as "baby steps to success." While these steps need to be made relevant to anything you want to master, it does help you to see mastery as a process or a journey.

The four stages to mastery:

1. **Unconsciously incompetent**

2. **Consciously incompetent**

3. **Consciously competent**

4. **Unconsciously competent**

The best way to understand this concept is through a simple example familiar to most of us: learning to ride a bike.

When you are three years old, you are *unconsciously incompetent* when it comes to riding a bike. At that age, most have not thought about riding a bike or even experimented.

At six or seven, you get you your first bike. You get on it and fall. While you strongly want to learn to ride, you don't yet think it will happen. You are *consciously incompetent.*

After some scrapes and bruises, you finally begin to get your balance. You are actually riding. You may not ride well, but you are entering stage three of mastery (*consciously competent*). While you are happy that you have accomplished this, you find it stressful and not a very relaxing riding experience. You're spending a lot of mental energy just trying not to fall off the bike.

After many hours of riding and practice you begin to move into stage four of mastery, when you become *unconsciously competent.* You don't have to think about being able to ride. You now can experiment with some riding tricks. You now begin to enjoy the view. You now can have a comfortable conversation with someone riding with you. All these are early stage-four mastery experiences. Now you really begin to see the return on the investment of learning and mastering bike riding.

I share this simple analogy because it is parallel to the higher levels of time mastery. If you want to see the maximum returns in time mastery you need to become a student of success. You need to become so proficient at the system and the subject that you become *unconsciously competent* at planning your day. When you reach this level, you not only automatically and gracefully use the system, but you can go much deeper and find answers to questions and ways to be more effective.

As much as I would like to give you a magic pill to get there, it really just takes three things:

> **Commitment:** If you lose the commitment to master time you will fall off the wagon and fail.
>
> **Focus:** You need to stay laser-focused on improving your skills every day.
>
> **Capital:** It requires an investment of time to gain time mastery.

Generally, after about thirty days, you can reach level three of mastery, but level four is a continuous improvement process. The reason you want to push, however, is so you can continue to gain time-mastery insights and benefit (ROI) year after year. People who reach the fourth level of mastery gain hundreds of hours a year of more effective time. They are less stressed, and they accomplish more.

They keep promises and exceed expectations. Overall they feel better and more fulfilled.

Try to think in terms of baby steps. Be patient with yourself. Don't forget to celebrate the progress as you continue to find the energy and discipline to get there.

# TIME MYTHS

**I need to wear a watch.** This is not true if it is for telling the time. Many years ago, my wife bought me a new watch. After about five years, the band broke. I took it to the jeweler, who said the cost to fix the band was as much as the watch itself. So I did not get it fixed and stopped wearing a watch until I could replace it. At first I was uncomfortable not always being able to check the time. I thought I would run late. But after a month or so, I had trained my brain to be sensitive to the time and could predict it very accurately. This is a skill/muscle, not magic. This is all about being in the moment and being in touch with time. When I am in a meeting or on a conference call, my body tells me when I am getting close to sixty minutes or when it is about 1:00 p.m. Again, it sounds a little mystical, but I know others who have also developed these skills.

## MASTERY TIPS

A famous architect (Mies van der Rohe) said, "God is in the details." This is definitely true when it comes to mastering time. After you have the blocking and tackling down in the system, then there are some tips that increase the effectiveness and where you can see increased returns.

The following are my top-ten tips to master the TMS:

### 1. Ask great questions during the planning process.

And know the important answers on a subconscious level.

     a.   Why am I doing this?

     b.   Is there another way to accomplish it?

     c.   How can I leverage this or expand the return?

By simply asking, you will find the plan will be more meaningful. You will find five or ten minutes here and there that add up to thirty to sixty minutes of dividend in the day.

### 2. Fill the page.

This system is designed to be done on an 8.5" x 11" notebook because that should represent a full day's worth of brain-dump activities (see examples). If your brain dump is only filling half of the page, go deeper. Add smaller items (a call or a few notes) that, when accomplished, can make a difference between a good day and a great one.

### 3. Confirm.

I like to send out quick confirmations in the morning in the first time slot (or before) regarding the meetings or calls that I am planning on. It is good to confirm what you expect. Otherwise your day gets thrown off by people forgetting, canceling, or running late

### 4. Use X when you are not sure.

As you are hooking the timeline into the brain-dump items, you want to match a letter with the time slot. However, these are filler items that really could be done in just about any time slot. I recommend using X. Then as you are moving through your day, either lock these in at particular slots—or just knock them out as you see fit. The win is getting it done, not fitting it into the correct time slot.

### 5. Bounce around.

After you have the basic process down (where you are consciously competent), you might find there are benefits on some days to bouncing the order of the steps around a little. For example, if I am feeling like the day is crammed, I might go ahead and begin a rough timeline so I can visualize my day before I get too deep into my brain dump. I might also go to the other tools that are highlighted in the "taking it to the next level" chapter, like the stress cloud,[1] which may influence what I want my activities to be that day or how aggressive I want to be. Over time you will find this process is very meditative, so you might wander a bit, as long as you end up with an end plan for the day.

---

1    *See explanation on page 136.*

## 6. Leverage the gaps.

Often what makes a day great is the little things you accomplish, not just the big to-do items. As you are analyzing the rough design (before launch), try to focus on the gaps. The gaps are the time between things. It could be fifteen minutes between meetings or calls, or it could be the time to drive twenty minutes to get to an appointment. I generally will hit five to fifteen small actions/add-ons a day in these gaps. But the key is to plan them. You may want to give some of these an X time slot, if you have multiple gaps.

## 7. Master world-class voicemails.

I know voicemails can be annoying and frustrating, but they are an excellent time-mastery tool if done well. When you are doing your morning planning, ask yourself if a voicemail may be an efficient way to communicate. If the answer is yes, then plan for it. If you want to leave a voicemail, the best time to do it is when you know the other person won't be answering the call (a time of day while they are in a meeting or at the gym). Jot down a little outline of what you want to communicate. Make the message concise, but complete enough. Then send a text or e-mail saying you left a "lengthy" voicemail and ask for a reply. You can save twenty to thirty minutes a day by doing this sort of world-class voicemailing. And that can add up to sixty hours a year. This does take a little practice and preparation, but the key is to begin to plan them, not just react when the other person does not answer his or her phone.

## 8. Multitask.

Our ability to multitask today is greater than ever. The speed at which our brains must process is faster. Our ability to do two or three things at once competently is better. It is critical that you are uber-focused when you need to be, but you can also plan to do more than one thing during some activities. Again, once you have mastered the basic planning system, then ask yourself during the morning planning session if they are activities that can be done while doing something else. These, by the way, may be personal, too. For example, you can clean up e-mails when on a group conference call, or you can sit outside and get fresh air to recharge during a call, or you can walk your dog and talk on the phone.

**9. Invest in the tools.**

There are many simple technology tools that can make things easier. Here are a few I use:

a. Using a wireless headset for calls allows me to move about and do other simple tasks while on calls. This saves me twenty minutes a day, which equals sixty hours a year.

b. I use a phone camera to text/e-mail images.

c. The voice recorder on the phone allows me to record text/e-mail messages. I find these little recordings are a great way to communicate effectively. Then I blast them out to the recipient(s).

d. Get yourself a high-quality day timer. It must have extra pages for your additional planning tools and a pocket in the back for goal-tracking tools and other important information. I religiously carry one of these around all the time, so I chose one that looks presentable when I pull it out. I find this to be an important tool for planning.

**10. Set up a mobile office.**

While safe driving is always the top priority, you can also leverage your time in the car. Here are three ways to use/think of your mobile office:

1. **It's a communication command center.** Make sure you have all the tools, both high tech and high touch.

2. **It's a mobile university.** This is a great training opportunity; listen to podcasts, training CDs, books, etc.

3. **It's a think tank.** Use this time for deeper reflection on important things that require some meditativeness. Make a list of questions you want to ask yourself while driving.

If you know you are going to be in your car for commuting or for chunks of time during the day or week, then really make it a priority to plan in these gaps of times. Doing this also gives you greater freedom when you know the office is mobile and you can accomplish many things on the move.

# TIME MYTHS

**An appointment means it's going to happen.** An appointment is just a placeholder until it is confirmed. Think how many times appointments have been postponed or cancelled. Then just multiply the amount of time this would waste. It represents hundreds of hours in a year. If you can be disciplined about not assuming a meeting or appointment is going to happen unless you confirm it, you will increase your effectiveness substantially. Adding this proactivity to your thinking will save time and make you more effective.

# TAKING IT TO THE NEXT LEVEL

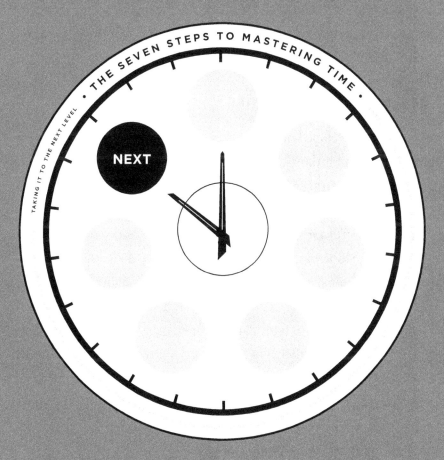

*Practice makes perfect.*

UNKNOWN

**A**fter you have gotten to stage three of mastery and you are beginning to enter stage four (*unconsciously competent*), you can begin to weave in other planning tools and techniques to increase your mastery of time and your success. Some of these "taking it to the next level" tools have been developed to look at time from a different angle and in different intervals. While you will be able to benefit from these, I also encourage you to now begin to get a little more creative and use this methodology to customize and develop your own tools. While I continue to be a very low-tech person, I recognize that by leveraging technology you may also gain a few insights and efficiency in your day.

## ANNUAL/QUARTERLY PLANNING

One tool I developed and use is a tool for medium- or longer-term planning. I call it the T-9 (Top 9) tool.

The idea of this tool comes from my annual planning process. At the end of every year I take two or three days to plan the following year. (You don't have to wait until the end of the year to do this.) This is sort of like hibernating for three days and is a personal/professional strategic-planning process. I generally begin by doing a deep-dive inventory. This is where I think about and reflect on the previous year. I try to drill into hard data and metrics as well as feelings and emotions. I try to solicit input from my personal and professional circles of influence. Over the years I have found that the best way to take this inventory is in specific categories rather than in one big bite. I have found that nine to ten categories work best to yield goals and actions that I can monitor effectively.

The categories I use are:

1.  My health (physical/mental/emotional)

2. My wife

3. My family

4. My friends/relationships

5. My home

6. My financials

7. My fun/fulfillment

8. My work

9. My community

You can certainly add or delete from this list, but I find nine a good number of categories. For a visualization of the T-9 tool, see page 132.

**The process:**

1. Think about a few overriding themes for the year that touch most of the categories. These can be a product of where you are now, something you want to change, or something you want to continue doing. These themes are the glue that touches most of the categories. Some of my themes for the year I wrote this book (2017):

   a. Balance

   b. Time is the key

   c. Be thirsty

   d. Good health = +++

   e. Avoid mistakes

   f. Say no, too

# THE T-9 TOOL

| ANNUAL THEMES | Balance • Time Is the Key • Be Thirsty | | |
|---|---|---|---|
| Themes | 1st Quarter | 2nd Quarter | Annual Goals |
| **Health**<br>Age Well<br>Be Active<br>Gain Knowledge | Lose five pounds by cutting back on dessert/drinking<br>Doctor's appt. | | Weight to 185 lbs.<br>Bike to beach<br>Develop a new hobby |
| **Wife** | | | |
| **Family** | | | |
| **Relationships** | | | |
| **Home** | | | |
| **Financials** | | | |
| **Fulfillment** | | | |
| **Professional**<br>Stay relevant<br>20% fresh<br>Authority | Book manuscript 90%<br>Invest more time in Harvard | | Write two books<br>Create Remodeling Mastery Boot Camp |
| **Community** | | | |

2. Then for each subcategory have some subthemes:

    a. Health category themes:

        i. Age well

        ii. Be active

        iii. Gain knowledge

    b. For the professional category:

        i. Stay relevant

        ii. 20% fresh

        iii. Authority

While I think these themes are important, they just need to give direction. They are not the actions or necessarily the goal.

3. The next steps are to establish the actions for each. Begin with some annual goals for each category. For example:

    a. Health:

        i. Weight to 185 lbs.

        ii. Bike to beach

        iii. Develop a new hobby

    b. Professional:

        i. Write two books

        ii. Create Remodeling-Mastery Boot Camp

        iii. Write one more monthly column/blog

4. With these overarching themes and the individual subthemes in mind, try to come up with three to five actions in the first quarter for each. For example, for the

category of health and the previous themes (age well / be active / gain knowledge), the first quarter actions are:

a. Lose five pounds by cutting back on dessert/drinking.

b. Avg. 4 x week of 30 to 60 min. of exercise.

c. Dr. apt for a check up.

d. Travel well (pack to eat / exercise).

e. Get a DNA test.

For the professional category:

a. Book manuscript 90%.

b. Avg. 40 hours per week with clients.

c. Deeper magazine relationship.

d. Invest more time in Harvard.

e. Move Thought-Leaders program forward.

I generally prefer to have a detailed next quarter and a loose following quarter (it gets readjusted on a monthly basis).

After you have this road map, you need a system to monitor it. I generally like to do a sixty- to ninety-minute-deep daily plan every Monday. In this additional time, I review the top-nine areas of my life, or my T-9 (and the other following tools). I ask myself how I can move these actions in my day and week. I reflect on the themes to make sure I continue to have my priorities right.

You can really take it to the next level with this simple tool.

## GOAL-SETTING TOOL

### *A goal without a plan is just a wish.*

ANTOINE DE SAINT-EXUPÉRY

There are many goal-setting tools that you can use, but I have learned over the years that none will work unless it is:

1.  **Meaningful.** Really thought through both in importance and realistic timing.

2.  **Concise.** I have had short ones and long ones, but the ones I can review and think about easily are the best. By the way, you may have mountains of back-up data/thoughts/ notes, but what you look at regularly needs to be concise (ideally one page).

3.  **In bite-size pieces.** You can't eat a pizza in one bite. By breaking goals into parts both in categories and in time frames, you can think through and really focus

So, with all that said, I like to begin with a simple spreadsheet or list using my T 9 categories.

I then like to list a few long-term (three- to five-year) goals for each. It is important that you take into account how time changes for other people involved (e.g., if one of the goals is that you want to take your kids on a cross-country trip, then keep in mind that—if they are ten and twelve years old now—in five years they will be fifteen and seventeen and may not be interested in going on the trip with you).

I encourage you to list the stretch goals. Try to also write down the obstacles or potholes that would keep you from reaching this goal (like money, time, health etc.).

Then I try to narrow this down to three big goals from each category.

Next you want to move from five years, down to three, then down to the coming year.

Generally, this will result in just a few big goals for the year. I like to create a one-page chart with each of these goals. I can read on a weekly basis and ask myself: How can I inch this goal along this week? When should I lock this event or goal into my calendar (based on my other activities)? Is this goal still relevant and aggressive but realistic?

## STRESS CLOUDS

As you know by now, I am a visual thinker. I can communicate with words; however, if I can find a metaphor or a diagram to express a concept or an idea, then my level of mastery on the subject increases exponentially. I only began using this technique or tool a few years before this writing, but it has made a big difference in my ability to balance, control, and reduce my stress. Unlike some of the other tools, I only pull this one out when I need it (when I am feeling some overwhelm and stress). It is sort of like taking an aspirin when you have a headache.

The metaphor is what I call "stress clouds." On a bright, sunny day, there are no clouds in the sky versus a dark, dreary day when the cloud cover is so thick that you cannot see the sun at all. Needless to say, most days are in between, with a few clouds. Being a sun guy (as most people are) I feel better and more energized on the sunny days versus feeling sad and a little depressed on the no-sun days.

In your day or week, we all have stress clouds. Most can handle several small ones and still feel good. Some can handle one big one as long as there are not any little ones creeping in.

The purpose of this tool/exercise is to identify what these clouds are, how big they are, and what is needed to make them go away or vaporize.

The first step I take is to draw myself as a simple stick figure.

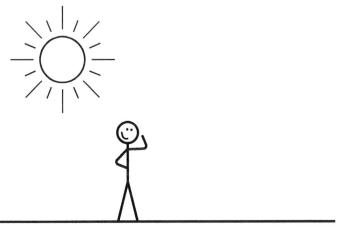

CLEAR SKIES

Then I begin to draw the clouds. The sizes or shapes vary depending on the level of stress that they are causing me. For example, if I have a big speaking presentation on a new topic in four days and I am not feeling like I have nailed it, I may draw a big cloud and write the name of the talk in it. If, on the other hand, I have the same presentation and I feel fully prepared but need to confirm a few details to finalize it, I will draw a little cloud.

Now, sticking to the metaphor, the big cloud blocks the sun more than the little one. I continue to create different clouds from different places (personal, health, relationship strain, and other projects to complete). What might be adding to the stress that I am feeling?

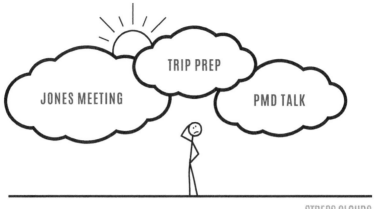

STRESS CLOUDS

Then I take a couple of minutes to look at the visual holistically. I ask myself, does this represent the stress that I am feeling? How would I feel if some of this stress were gone? Do I believe I can reduce these stress clouds? Is there someone else who can help me with this?

Then I write out two to five actions steps on a notebook page for each cloud that would shrink or vaporize the cloud.

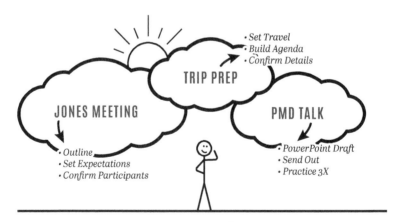

ACTIONS TO VAPORIZE STRESS CLOUDS

Then I keep this piece of paper with me as I am doing my daily planning. Generally, I cannot attack all the items on that day, or even in a couple of days, but I always feel better knowing that I am in control, and I recognize the stress is usually something that can be reduced quickly, if I take action.

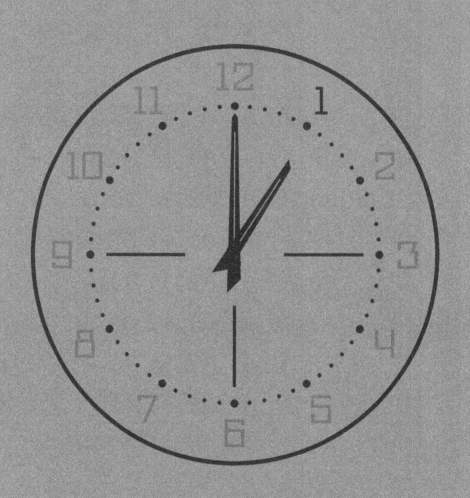

# IN CLOSING

......................................................

*Unexpressed good thoughts aren't worth squat!*

KEN BLANCHARD

Over the last twenty-five years, I have made huge strides in mastering my time. These are strides, not final destinations. These strides have given me real and meaningful returns. By sharing these insights and the time-management system, I hope you will be able to see the same returns in months, not years.

As I shared earlier in this book, the goal is to first focus on strong "whys," and they will give you the conviction to stick with the system.

The following are what you should expect to achieve:

- Reduce stress. (This may be the biggest benefit for many people.)

- Accomplish more.

- Stay on track with your goals and resolutions.

- Think more clearly.

- Look longer term.

- Keep important promises.

- Exceed expectations.

- Be more predictable.

- Have time for other priorities.

- Have control of your destiny.

How each person processes this material is very personal. Some of you may have found it interesting and will tuck away a nugget or two to use when it is relevant to you. Others will be back to your old habits and continue to feel the stress of having others control your day. (I hope when the pain is great enough you will remember to dust this off and revisit the advice I have shared.) Then there will be a handful of the students of success. You are the ones who embrace change, shift your thinking, and develop the habits to achieve the results.

Having taught these time-mastery techniques to thousands of people, I am not here to judge which group you fall into. I want you to be aware that being in control of your day is a *choice*. If you choose to take control, then this summary is just the beginning. The following are some further tips as you dive into this process.

1. It takes time to develop new habits, so be patient with yourself.

2. We all need a coach, so grab a friend or reach out to me if you need help.

3. Visualize and believe in the rewards of mastering time.

4.   If you fail to plan, then plan to fail.

5.   Tell others about your thirst to improve, and they will be your cheerleaders for success

This book is only one piece of the time-mastery jigsaw puzzle. It may be the centerpiece, but you should think about adding some of these other tools to be successful:

1.   Contact Mark G. Richardson for relevant links and access to the below.

2.   Watch the time-mastery video to see the actual techniques being done.

3.   Listen to the time-mastery audio, where I will walk you through these techniques and concepts.

4.   Check out the time-mastery webinar (a sixty-minute webinar to supplement your learning).

5.   Sign up for a time-mastery workshop (see the site for dates).

6.   Seek out one-on-one time coaching.

7.   Call the time-mastery "hotline."

Thank you. I wish you well in your journey to take control of your day and master your time!

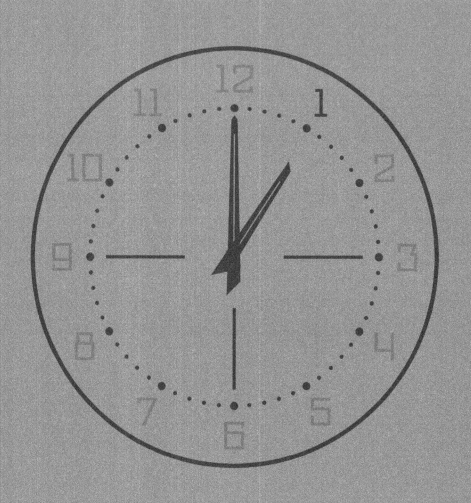

# ABOUT THE AUTHOR

MARK G. RICHARDSON's involvement in construction, design, and business spans more than three decades. A graduate of the School of Architecture at Virginia Tech, his career has been defined by leadership and an entrepreneurial spirit. As the former Co-Chairman and President of Case, he led the growth of over 1,000 percent by expanding services and market reach. For ten years he hosted "At Home with Mark Richardson," a weekly radio show dedicated to bringing a slice of the remodeling industry to consumers and practitioners alike. Mark's passion for teaching and speaking generally takes complex ideas and simplifies things for diverse groups.

Mark is a guest lecturer for MBA programs at Virginia Tech, Georgetown University, Maryland University, and George Washington University. He serves as a business advisor to many business sectors from small practices to major corporations. In 2007 he developed a series of online business workshops and videos designed to offer professional, effective, and intelligent business practices from business fitness to sales and marketing strategies.

Mark is a Sr. Fellow at Harvard University's Joint Center for Housing Studies and sits on many boards including Systems Pavers, N. Kelly Companies, Harrell, BBB, Revere Bank, and Advantage Media Group. He is also a regular columnist for *Professional Remodeler, Professional Builder,* and *Big Growers* magazines. Other Mark Richardson vehicles include: The Remodeling Thirty Day Fitness Program, Remodeling Live, and Business over Breakfast series. In 2006 Mark was named Entrepreneur of the Year with Ernst and Young. In 2008 Mark was inducted into the National Association of Home Builders Hall of Fame.

Mark continues to write, speak, and consult with diverse organizations in an effort to help them improve and grow. He can be reached at mrichardson@mgrichardson.com.

The Time Mastery System©
Mark G. Richardson
301.275.0208 | mrichardson@mgrichardson.com

# "A GIFT OF TIME"

## Time Mastery Workbook

**Mark G. Richardson**

mrichardson@mgrichardson.com

Printed in the USA
CPSIA information can be obtained
at www.ICGtesting.com
JSHW011602020424
60428JS00018B/707